Disclaimer: This textbook is not intended to provide, and disclaims any suggestion that it does provide, medical advice of any nature. The information made available through this textbook should not be used in place of seeking professional opinions by licensed practitioners. Only licensed medical professionals may offer medical advice, diagnosis and recommendations for treatment of medical conditions. You assume full responsibility for appropriate use of the information available through this textbook.

As Medicine is an ever-changing science, with new research and clinical experience, changes in treatment and techniques are required. The authorhas checked with sources believed to be reliable in effort to provide information that is complete and generally in accord with standards accepted at the time of publication. The opinions expressed in this work represent those of the author(s) and, in view of the possibility of human error or changes in medical science, neither the author(s), RAEducation.com LLC, nor any other party who has been involved in the preparation or publication of this work warrants that the information contained herein is in every respect accurate or complete and they are not responsible for any errors or omissions or for the results obtained from the use of such information. Readers and viewers are encouraged to confirm the information contained herein with other sources.

ISBN-10:   1-948083-03-5
ISBN-13:   978-1-948083-03-4

André P. Boezaart

MBChB, MPraxMed, DA(CMSA), FFA(CMSA), MMed(Anesth),
PhD
Professor of Anesthesiology and Orthopaedic Surgery
Chief of Division of Acute and Peri-operative Pain Medicine
Chief of Acute Pain Service
University of Florida College of Medicine,
Gainesville, Florida, USA

Artwork by:
Mary K. Bryson, MAMS, CMI
Bryson Biomedical Illustration
Langhorne, Pennsylvania
©2006

Educational electronic and printed media for the website
RAEducation.com owned by RAEducation.com LLC.

Please visit www.RAEducation.com
for video tutorials on this and other topics

Dedication

This book is dedicated to my late mother, Elma Boezaart,
who told me, as a small boy way back in 1956,
after I had a mastoidectomy,
that it was not necessary in "modern times" to suffer pain.
She did not know how far we still had to go,
yet she already understood that pain is half treated
if we merely acknowledge its existence.

Managing Acute Pain with Nerve Blocks

A GUIDE FOR PATIENTS

2nd Edition

Preface

The second edition of this booklet follows on the very successful first edition, published in 2005. The discipline of acute and perioperative pain medicine has undergone explosive growth over the past 12 to 18 years, with many older concepts now being replaced with more modern ideas. In addition, we also face new societal challenges – the opioid crisis being just one very disturbing example.

The purpose of this booklet is to provide patients with information about regional anesthesia. The author hopes that the information provided in this booklet will answer most of the questions that patients may have, but more importantly, that it will stimulate discussion between patients, surgeons and anesthesiologists.

With the advent of increased outpatient surgery, and more so that is done minimally invasive manner, the era of large doses of opioids and other potent and potentially dangerous drugs is drawing to a close. A larger contingent of surgeons and anesthesiologists are relying on single-injection and continuous nerve blocks to manage surgical and other acute pain.

After this book's Introduction, the reader can search for the type of surgery that he or she is scheduled for from the Table of Contents and read about the appropriate nerve blocks likely to be offered for this procedure and to manage postoperative pain. The specific blocks are color-coded to make referencing easy.

Patients are encouraged to discuss these regional anesthesia procedures with their anesthesiologists, surgeons, friends and colleagues. All the blocks and procedures described in this booklet can be viewed on www.RAEducation.com, which is free for patients.

André P. Boezaart, 2018

INTRODUCTION

This booklet is intended to provide information on nerve blocks (also known as regional anesthesia). Today, patients, surgeons, and anesthesiologists have more options than ever before for anesthesia and pain control after surgery than. Regional anesthesia is a proven, safe alternative to traditional pain management, and it provides superior pain control. In the following pages, you will find a description of the most common types of peripheral nerve blocks and you are encouraged to use this information when planning your surgery, anesthesia, and postoperative care.

Anesthesiologists are physicians who, in addition to putting you "to sleep" for surgery, specialize in preventing and relieving pain. Over the years, anesthesiologists have responded to the challenges posed by surgeons and patients to make anesthesia safe for longer and more complex surgery in more critically ill patients. Anesthesia is now safe; the next challenge is to make anesthesia user-friendly—that is, more user-friendly to society by making it and surgery more cost-effective, and more user-friendly to the individual patient by addressing the anxiety, nausea, vomiting, and pain associated with surgery. Anxiety is receiving high-quality attention at present, and the answer to avoiding nausea and vomiting, which have also received widespread research attention, centers mainly on avoiding general anesthesia and narcotics (like morphine) for pain management. Managing pain from surgery can be done very effectively with regional anesthesia and peripheral nerve blocks. If the surgical pain is eliminated from the equation, then anesthesia can be light, relatively free of side effects, and user-friendly, and opioids can be avoided to a large extent.

8   **What Is a Peripheral Nerve Block?**

Our nervous system is basically divided into three sections: the sensory, motor, and autonomic nervous systems. The brain and spinal cord comprise the central nervous system. Nerve cells outside the brain and spinal cord are peripheral nerves, which have the job of transmitting sensation and movement signals to and from the brain, and are protected by fluid-filled spaces along the spinal column and, farther out, by muscle or fat tissue. Bones forming the cranium and spinal column protect the brain and spinal cord. The tissues surrounding nerves play an important role in determining how much medication is used, how fast a block works, and how long a block will last.

A peripheral nerve block is the injection of anesthetic medications, similar to what a dentist uses to numb the jaw, near a peripheral nerve. Blocks work because they temporarily prevent the nerve from sending signals to and from the brain. The most common medications used for injection include local anesthetics, opioids, such as morphine, and non-steroidal anti-inflammatory drugs (NSAIDS). Local anesthetics include drugs like lidocaine, which is routinely used for dental procedures. Lidocaine does not last as long as newer drugs in this class, such as ropivacaine. Opioids are drugs like Demerol or morphine that work in a slightly different way to block pain perception in the brain. NSAIDS reduce or prevent the inflammation and swelling that often occurs after tissue injury or surgery.

Depending on the procedure and the patient's medical history, a combination of regional and general anesthesia may be used during surgery. Combining the two therapies allows the general anesthesia to be very light (meaning the patient will wake up much faster after surgery, but not during the surgery) and provides better pain control after surgery. In many cases, nerve blocks are performed along with a rehabilitation program that provide the patient with a window of opportunity for more effective recovery. Deciding to have a peripheral nerve block will not prevent patients from receiving additional pain medication, if needed. Medications to lessen a patient's anxiety, stress, and pain are routinely used during nerve block procedures and most patients have no recollection of the procedures. It is not painful or uncomfortable to undergo a nerve block procedure.

10   How Is a Peripheral Nerve Block Performed?

A peripheral nerve block can be performed as a single injection of medication or it may be a continuous infusion of medication for several days or weeks. The anesthesiologist will determine which nerve block is best for the patient. Discussions of the various types of nerve blocks are included in later pages. For single-injection nerve blocks in general, numbness may last 6 to 12 hours. Much longer numbness, up to 36 hours, is not uncommon for certain lower leg blocks. Patients should begin taking their prescribed pain medication before the block wears off. For example, patients should take their pain medication at bedtime after a morning surgery even if the extremity still feels numb and free of pain, or they should start taking their pain medication immediately when they feel sensation returning to the limb. This usually presents with a feeling of "pins-and-needles." Patients with obstructive sleep apnea (OSA) should discuss this with their anesthesiologists because OSA plus opioids may be a very dangerous combination, leading to a continuous nerve block as a much better choice. After surgery, CPAP machines are also mandatory for patients with OSA.

Soft, thin catheters placed next to nerves for continuous nerve blocks offer the advantage of more long-term pain relief. This type of therapy is also called "CPNB" or continuous peripheral nerve block. A small volume of anesthetic is dripped onto the nerve every second, and every 30 or 60 minutes, the patient can, if he or she requires it, press a button that will infuse a larger volume over a short period of time. This is what is known as "PCRA" or patient-controlled regional anesthesia." For this procedure, a thin catheter, or tube, the size of thick fishing line is inserted through a needle that has been placed through the skin after properly numbing the skin near the target nerve. The entry site for this catheter will depend on the particular nerve and the type of surgery to be performed. The various types of nerve blocks are discussed in the following pages. The catheter connects to a disposable pump about the size of a portable CD player. The catheter and pump are designed to provide an infusion of local anesthetic such as lidocaine or ropivacaine, all in the Novocain family, which provides pain relief for as long as the infusion runs. There is no need to worry about overdosing or receiving too much medication; the pump has built-in safety features to protect the patient.

The Food and Drug Administration, or FDA, is the federal agency responsible for approving drugs and devices safe for human use. The nerve block catheters currently available have FDA approval for up to 72 hours of use. Although it is safe to leave the catheter in for longer periods of time, this must be discussed with the anesthesiologist.

Nerve blocks are usually performed just before surgery in a dedicated Block Procedure Room. The patient's blood pressure and heart and breathing rates will be monitored closely throughout the procedure. Ultrasound, in combination with a small hand-held machine called a nerve stimulator, is routinely used during nerve block procedures. An ultrasound works on sound waves similar to the navigation systems of bats and dolphins and are safe and there is no sensation associated with its use. Pregnant women are all very familiar with sonar or ultrasound machines, as the ultrasounds used for nerve blocks are exactly the same as those used in obstetric practice. The nerve stimulator, on the other hand, sends a low-level electrical signal into the tissue below the skin and helps to pinpoint the precise nerve location. The signal triggers brief muscle contractions, like an eye twitch. The patient may experience minor discomfort from the muscle contractions, but the sensation will be very brief and 99% of patients are not bothered by these. Some patients may even find the twitch sensation amusing. Depending on individual needs, medication may be given to help patients relax. If the nerve block is being performed for treatment of a painful condition like a broken arm or leg, medications will be given to prevent pain. Under certain circumstances, such as in children or very anxious people, the procedure can be performed while the patient is under heavy sedation or asleep with general anesthesia.

12   Side Effects & Potential Complications

Almost every procedure a physician performs has the potential for side effects or complications. In the case of nerve blocks this risk is extremely low, and the anesthesiologists take every precaution to prevent these. To prevent complications, patients should also inform their anesthesiologist about any problems they or a member of their family have had with anesthesia, including any at the dentist's office. Important information to share with the doctor includes:

- Any allergies or side effects to drugs
- Any medication taken in the last four weeks, including herbal supplements
- Any bleeding disorder, frequent bruising with minor injuries, or recurrent nose bleeds
- Any medical condition involving heart, lung, kidney, or liver function; nervous system or psychiatric problems; or the metabolic system (like diabetes, thyroid problems, or genetic disease)
- Repeated pressure neuropathies, such as carpal tunnel release in the patient or his/her family
- Existing numbness or "pins-and-needles" in a limb

With either single-injection or continuous nerve blocks, it is important that patients report any unusual sensations to their doctor, especially at the start of the block procedure. This includes a metallic taste in the mouth, a ringing in the ears, or other hearing or visual sensations. Patients should also report any feelings of anxiety or muscle spasms. Problems like a reduction in blood pressure or heart rate from the injection of local anesthetics are usually easy to treat. Severe side effects that require resuscitation are extremely rare, and are most often associated with severe pre-existing illness.

Bleeding and infection at the nerve block puncture site are rare but potential complications. A thorough review of the patient's medical history, a physical examination, and a discussion of medications (including non-prescription and herbal drugs) by the doctor will minimize these potential dangers. The nerve block procedure will be done using an aseptic technique, which simply means the doctor will take the necessary steps to minimize the risk of infection.

Long surgical procedures sometimes result in temporary nerve damage, especially to arms and legs. Slender individuals and elderly people are at greater risk for this potential complication. Position-related nerve damage happens despite careful padding of potential pressure points and observation during surgery. Position-related nerve damage usually resolves in a few weeks or months and is not related to the regional block used. A peripheral nerve block resulting in permanent damage to the nerve is very rare. The surgery itself, especially shoulder surgery, may also cause temporary nerve injury – usually because of traction on the arm during surgery.

As with all medications, the drugs used for peripheral nerve blocks can cause allergic reactions or unpleasant side effects. Opioids like morphine can cause constipation, difficulty urinating, itching, nausea, and vomiting, and breathing problems, and the side effect profile of these drugs is the very reason for the existence of regional anesthesia and nerve blocks. If opioids were safe and effective without side effects, of which addiction is a very real problem, there would be no need for nerve blocks. The side effects of opioids, however, are often dose related; the more patients receive, the more likely they are to experience unpleasant side effects.

Patients should not drive or operate any machinery in the first 24 hours after a nerve block or for as long as they feel a residual block effect like numbness or weakness. This is especially the case with CPNBs.

14   Being "Awake" for the Operation

In the past, it was customary to give patients a choice between being "awake" or "asleep" for their surgery, i.e., having the surgery under regional anesthesia or peripheral nerve block only, or having the surgery under general anesthesia. This is no longer the case. With modern techniques and drugs, the patient can be anywhere between wide awake and totally unconscious. The choice is the patient's: as long as the pain of surgery is completely eliminated by the nerve block, the entire spectrum of consciousness is available to the patient. The medications used for sedation can make patients totally unaware of the procedure, but if they so choose, they may also be fully awake and aware of everything that is going on. If patients choose to be fully awake (the vast minority of patients), it is important for them to realize that the members of the surgical team need to concentrate on the task at hand and this is not the time for "small talk" or for questions for the surgeon. The surgeon will be more than happy to answer all questions after the surgery.

Which Block Is Likely To Be Offered?

The chart on the following pages gives you an idea of the block(s) that are most common for surgical procedures in specific areas of the body and a reference to the page upon which that block is described in this booklet.

Which Block is likely to be offered?

Planned Surgery	Likely Block	Page
Upper Limb		
Shoulder Surgery	Cervical paravertebral block	33
	Interscalene block	29
Elbow Surgery	Cervical paravertebral block	33
	Supraclavicular block	43
	Infraclavicular block	43
	Axillary block	47
Wrist Surgery	Cervical paravertebral block	33
	Supraclavicular block	43
	Infraclavicular block	43
	Axillary block	47
Upper Arm Surgery	Cervical paravertebral block	33
	Supraclavicular block	43
	Infraclavicular block	43
Lower Arm Surgery	Cervical paravertebral block	33
	Supraclavicular block	43
	Infraclavicular block	43
	Axillary block	47
Hand Surgery	Cervical paravertebral block	33
	Supraclavicular block	43
	Infraclavicular block	43
	Axillary block	47
	Elbow block	51
Lower Limb		
Hip Surgery	Spinal block	19
	Epidural block	23
	Lumbar paravertebral block	33
	Femoral nerve block	61
Knee Surgery	Spinal block	19
	Epidural block	23
	Lumbar paravertebral block	33
	Sciatic nerve block	55
	Femoral nerve block	61

16

Chart continued on next page

Planned Surgery	Likely Block	Page
Lower Limb (continued)		
Ankle Surgery	Sciatic nerve block	55
	Femoral nerve block	61
Foot Surgery	Sciatic nerve block	55
	Femoral nerve block	61
	Ankle block	65
Upper Leg Surgery	Spinal block	19
	Epidural block	23
	Lumbar paravertebral block	33
	Sciatic nerve block	55
	Femoral nerve block	61
Lower Leg Surgery	Sciatic nerve block	55
	Femoral nerve block	61
Chest Surgery		
Both sides	Thoracic epidural block	23
	Thoracic paravertebral block	33
Open Heart Surgery	Thoracic epidural block	23
Abdominal Surgery		
Midline	Spinal block (lower abdomen)	19
	Thoracic epidural block (upper)	23
	Lumbar epidural block (lower)	23
Unilateral	Epidural block	23
	Thoracic paravertebral block	33
	Lumbar paravertebral block	33
Caesarean Section	Spinal block	19
	Epidural block	23
	Combined spinal/epidural (CSE)	19 / 23
Gynecological	Spinal block	19
	Epidural block	23
Urological Surgery	Spinal block	19
	Epidural block	23

Note: All these blocks are also available for children.

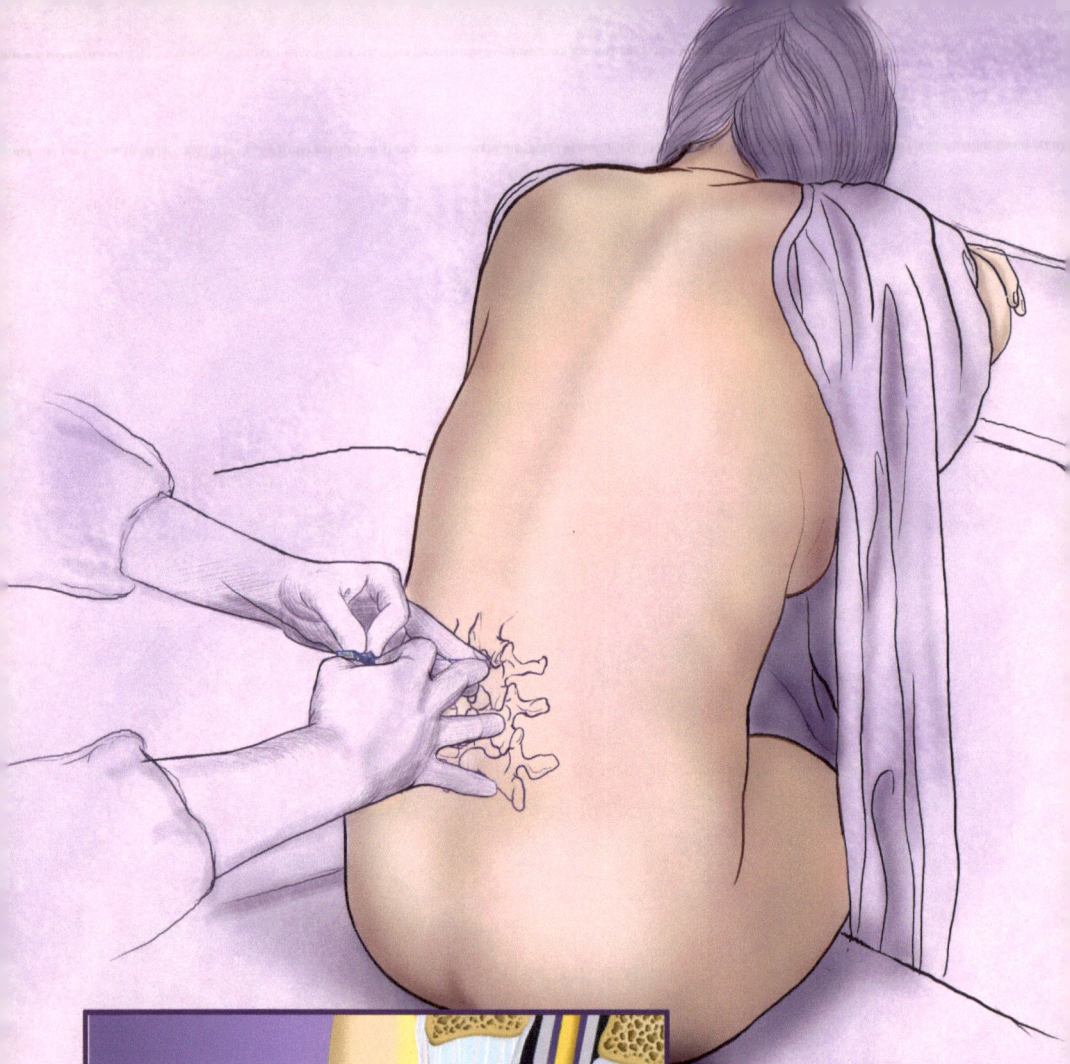
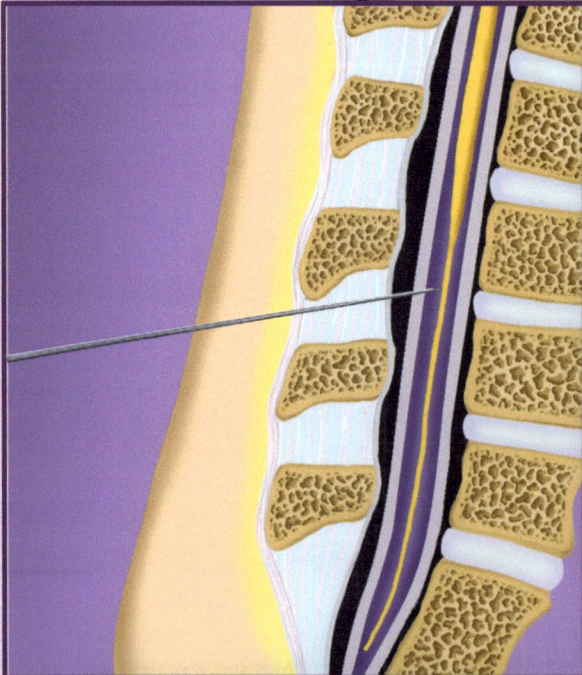

BRYSON©

Spinal Anesthesia

[Spinal Blocks, Subarachnoid Block
(sub = under or deep to; arachnoid is one of the membranes
surrounding the spinal cord)]

Spinal anesthesia dates back to 1899 and remains one of the most commonly used types of nerve block. Spinal blocks are frequently used for hernia repairs, surgery in the lower abdomen (such as prostate surgery and cesarean section), and for knee or hip surgery.

FIGURE 1:
Spinal anesthetic with patient seated.
Note: Needle is deep to membrane
surrounding spinal cord.

In adults, the nerve fibers that comprise the spinal cord come to an end about midway down the back; the remaining space is filled with a liquid called cerebrospinal fluid. The technique used for spinal anesthesia takes advantage of this fluid-filled space at the bottom of the spinal cord. Local anesthetics injected into the space produce numbness from about the waist down. For this procedure, the patient is asked to lie on her side or to sit. Body position is very important with this type of block and is dependent on the type of surgery to be performed. The anesthesiologist will give the patient specific instructions. Spinal procedures begin with carefully cleansing an area of skin on the lower back. A very small needle is then used to inject numbing medication into the skin and underlying tissue. It feels like a gentle pinch. With the area now numb to sensation, the rest of the procedure is painless. Through the numbed area, another fine needle is then inserted into the fluid-filled space of the spinal cord. Local anesthetic will be injected to provide complete numbness of the lower part of the body. The level of anesthesia can be slightly modified by positioning (head up or down). Depending on the medication and dose, a spinal block can provide pain relief after surgery for several hours.

What Are the Risks of Spinal Anesthesia?

Less than 1% of people who receive spinal anesthesia develop a "postural headache" following this procedure. Also called a postdural puncture headache, or PDPH, these headaches are worse when sitting or standing, and are relieved by lying flat in bed. The exact cause of this type of headaches is thought to be related to the tiny hole created in the tissue surrounding the fluid-filled space and cerebrospinal fluid leaking into the epidural space. With conservative treatment and bed rest, the headache usually goes away within 48 hours. If the pain persists, a "blood patch" treatment to seal the hole almost always relieves the pain. This involves injecting some of the patient's own blood near the hole.

Temporary pain in the lower back at the needle entry site or in the buttocks region can also occur. This discomfort is usually minor and resolves within a few days.

Difficulty passing urine is one of the more common problems because a spinal block also numbs the nerves controlling the bladder. This problem will disappear completely as the block wears off, but it is important to know how much urine is in the bladder at all times. The recovery room nurses will measure the volume in your bladder regularly with a bladder scan, and if a volume large enough to damage the bladder is present, it may be necessary to insert a tube (catheter) into the bladder to briefly relieve pressure and pass urine. Signs of this problem include an increase in heart rate and or blood pressure, and a feeling of pressure and/or pain below the waist.

Permanent damage to the spinal cord resulting in paralysis is extremely rare and is usually related to other severe complications like bleeding or infection. Permanent nerve injury occurs in approximately 1 of every 250,000 people receiving spinal anesthesia.

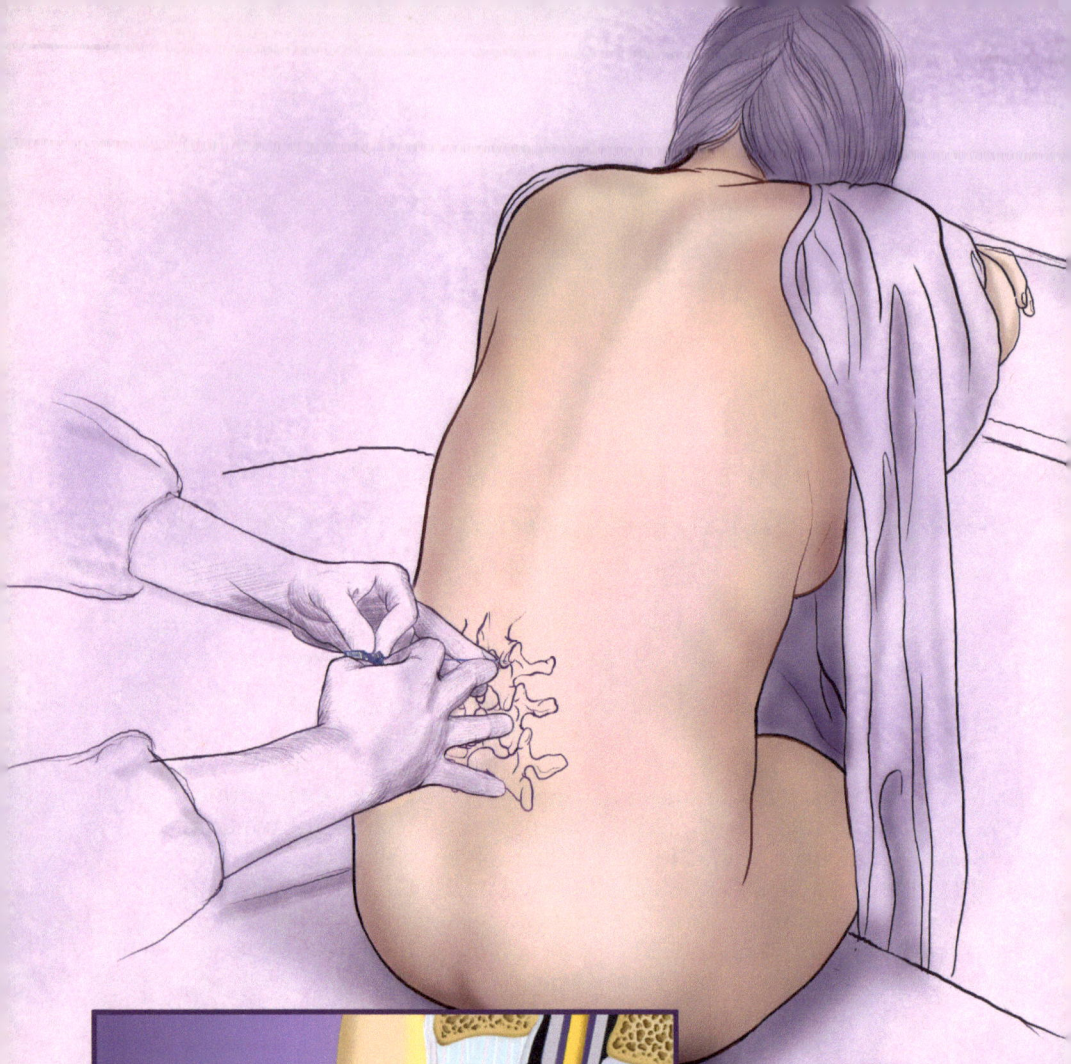

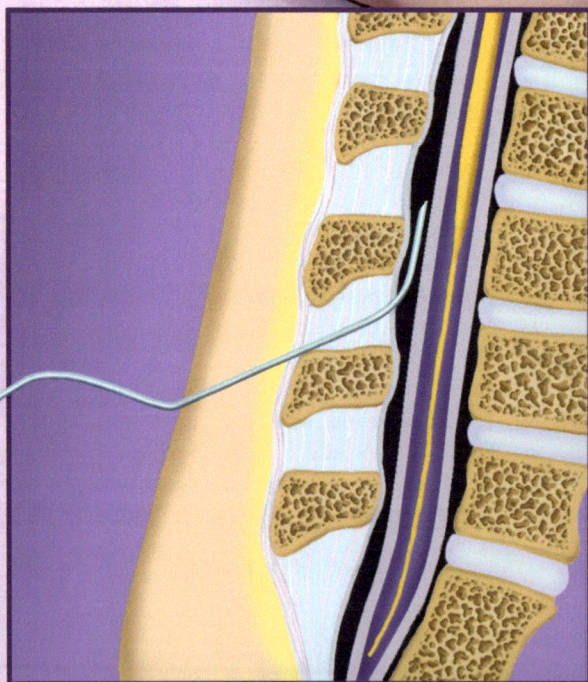

Epidural Anesthesia
(Epidural Blocks)
[(epi = outside; dura = the membrane surrounding fluid and the spinal cord)]

Epidural anesthesia is also a very common procedure, especially in the labor and delivery area where it is used to relieve the pain associated with childbirth. An epidural is like a spinal block, but the injection goes outside the membrane (the dura) surrounding the spinal cord. Epidural anesthesia requires more medication than spinal anesthesia and takes longer to reach full effect. The needle insertion point may be in the lower back (lumbar region) or upper back (thoracic region) and depends on the planned surgery.

FIGURE 2:
*Lumbar epidural with patient seated.
Note that the catheter is outside of the
membrane that surrounds the spinal cord.*

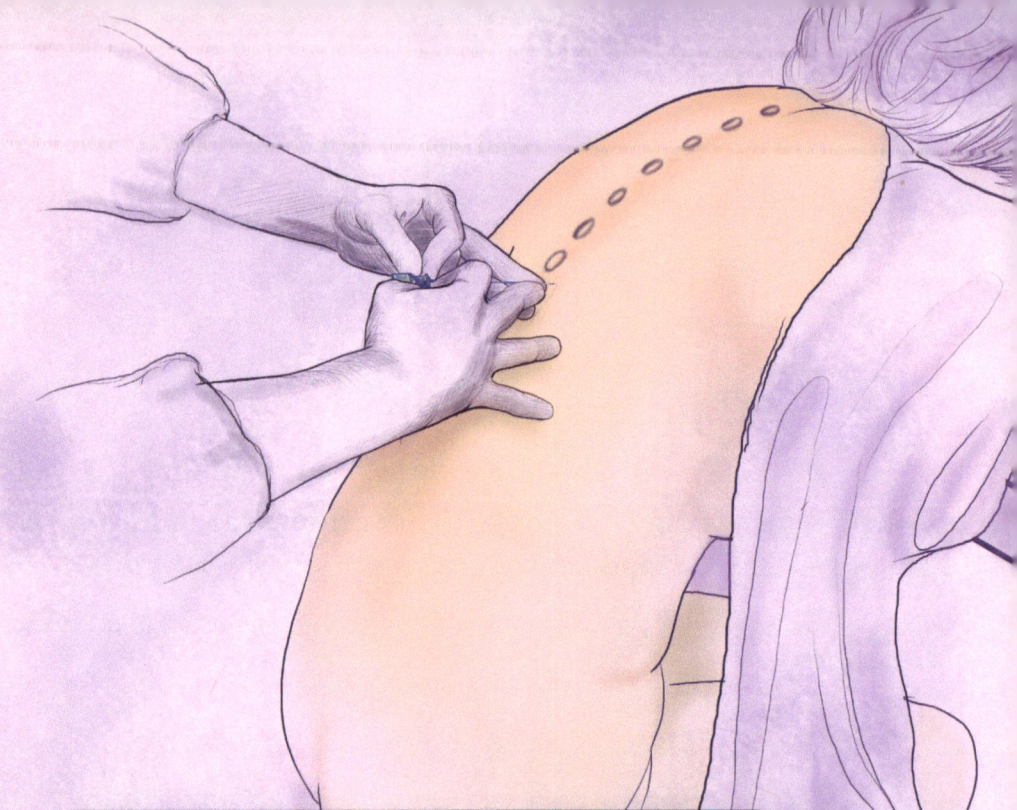

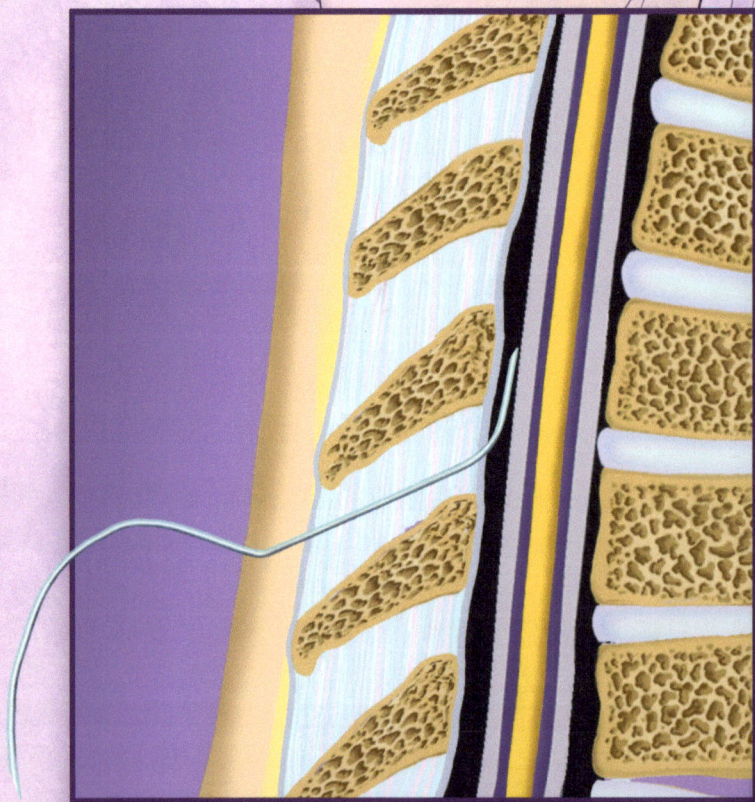

As with spinal anesthesia, the patient will be asked to lie on side or to sit. The skin around the needle entry site will be cleaned with an antiseptic soap. After the skin and tissues under the skin are numbed thoroughly with a very thin needle, a small plastic tube, the size of thick fishing line, will be inserted into the epidural space surrounding the spinal cord and fluid compartment. The patient may feel pressure in the area of the needle insertion, but no pain.

Epidural anesthesia allows the anesthesiologist to numb an area of the body most beneficial for the planned surgery. Voluntary movement is often lost as the epidural block begins to work. This means that patients may temporarily not be able to walk, or will need assistance walking. In modern practice, however, epidurals are "segmental," which means that only the segment being targeted is numbed. For example, if the surgery is in the abdominal area, only the belly can be numbed so that the legs, chest, and arms are not affected and the patient can ambulate (Figure 2b). The level can be selected to be anywhere where the planned surgery (and thus pain) is expected to be.

FIGURE 2B:
Thoracic epidural with patient seated.
Note that the catheter is outside of the
membrane that surrounds the spinal cord.

Epidural blocks can be a single injection of medication (usually a steroid injection for chronic back pain) or continuous. For the continuous infusion, the anesthesiologist will "fine-tune" the effect of the local anesthetics and other medication to provide pain relief with as little impairment of the patient's ability to walk as possible. The patient should not stand up or walk alone while the epidural infusion is in place. A healthcare provider should assess a patient's ability to move his or her arms and legs before making any attempt to stand or walk.

Sometimes, if a faster onset of the block is required, such as with childbirth and in emergency situations, a combined spinal and epidural block can be done—the combined spinal/epidural, or CSE. With this block, an epidural needle is first placed, and a thin spinal needle is then placed through this needle through the membrane that surrounds the spinal cord (the dura) and into the fluid surrounding the spinal cord. A small amount of local anesthetic agent is then injected through this needle, which causes an immediate onset of the block. An epidural catheter is then advanced through the same needle into the epidural space to be used for long-term infusion of a local anesthetic agent. This is done because the duration of a typical spinal block is relatively short-lived—2 to 5 hours at best. The CSE is only available for lower back or lumbar blocks because of the presence of the spinal cord higher up. Like regular spinals, it cannot be done above the level of the second lumbar vertebra because the spinal cord reaches that point and can be injured.

Risks with Epidural Anesthesia 27

Specific complications and side effects of epidural anesthesia include a so-called "wet tap." This means the needle accidentally penetrated the membrane around the spinal cord (the dura) and has entered the fluid-filled space. The anesthetic can then be continued as a spinal or it can be abandoned. Because a larger needle is used for epidural anesthesia than for planned spinal anesthesia, the incidence of headache after a wet tap may be higher than for spinal anesthesia. Under very rare circumstances, a larger volume of local anesthetic agent may accidentally be injected into the fluid-filled space, and a decrease in blood pressure or heart rate, or problems with breathing, can occur (the "total spinal"). If this occurs, general anesthesia will be required for the surgical procedure. This complication is also limited to the duration of the effects of the used local anesthetic—usually 2 to 3 hours. It is, however, extremely rare.

As is the case with spinal anesthesia, difficulty urinating can occur. A tube or catheter can be inserted into the bladder to drain urine. Urinary catheters are routinely used in patients scheduled for long surgical procedures and can also be used in patients planning to have an epidural catheter over a long period of time, but this is not always necessary because of the segmental nature of the epidural block, as explained above.

The risk of infection, although rare, increases with time as the epidural catheter is left in. Patients should report immediately to a nurse or physician any back pain, discharge from the puncture site, fever, or weakness or numbness not explained by a recent injection of local anesthetic.

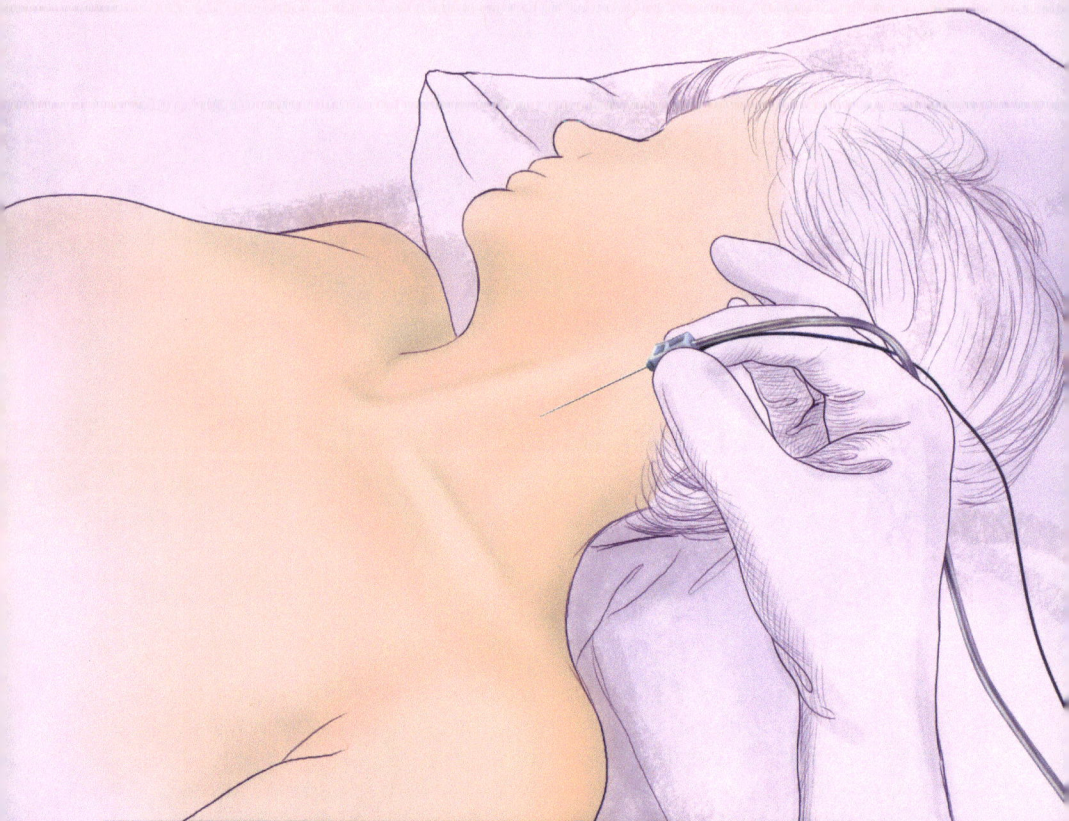

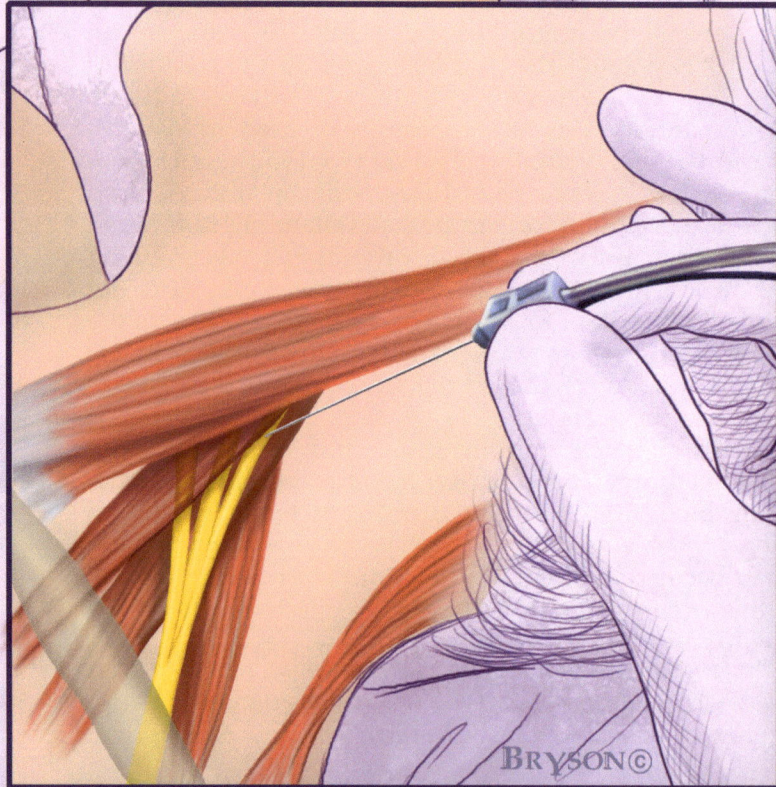

BRYSON©

Interscalene Blocks
[(inter = between;
scalene muscles = two muscles in the neck)]

29

An interscalene block is usually performed for shoulder surgery. This means that the block is placed on the front side of the lower neck, right above the collarbone. Patients are asked to lie flat on their back or in a semi-sitting position for the procedure, with the head turned slightly away from the side being blocked. The anterior and middle scalene muscles intersect on the right and left sides of the neck; the intersection of these muscles marks the location of several nerves supplying the upper arm. Patients are asked to lift their head slightly off the pillow at the start of the procedure to highlight these important surface landmarks; they are also sometimes asked to lie on their side for this block and the head of the bed is elevated 45 degrees.

FIGURE 3:
*Interscalene block.
Patient is supine with the head slightly
tilted to the other side.*

This block is typically done with ultrasound guidance. An antiseptic soap will be used to clean the skin in the area of the block. Sterile towels or drapes will be placed on the patient's skin to provide a clean working area for the doctor. A very fine needle will be used to inject local anesthetic into the skin and underlying tissue. This procedure should not be uncomfortable or painful as the local anesthetic will quickly numb the area, making the rest of the procedure pain-free. After the skin anesthetic, the anesthesiologist will use a specialized type of needle to perform the interscalene block. Patients may feel a little pressure at the needle insertion point, but no pain. The block may also be performed with nerve simulator guidance or both ultrasound and nerve stimulator guidance; known

as the dual technique, which seems to be the most popular approach. If a nerve stimulator is used, patients may detect a twitching of the muscles on the side that the block is done, mainly the biceps or triceps muscles. This is normal and should not be uncomfortable.

If a single injection of medication is planned for the interscalene block, the procedure ends after the local anesthetic is injected. For a continuous infusion, a very fine catheter will be threaded through the needle and secured in place with special tape applied to the skin. Most anesthesiologists also tunnel the catheter under the skin to prevent it from falling out. The needle is withdrawn, leaving only the very fine flexible tube. The tube connects to a small, disposable pump.

What Are the Risks of Interscalene Blocks?

The side effects associated with this block are related to numbing the other nerves of the arm, shoulder, and neck. Horner's syndrome is a temporary condition after an interscalene block in which individuals have unequal pupils and sometimes a slight drooping of one eyelid. People sometimes also get mild hoarseness from this type block, which happens because a branch of the nerve running to the vocal cords is numbed as well. Patients might also experience the feeling of a stuffy nose. Although unwanted, these are the usual effects of a working nerve block and not dangerous complications. They will wear off as soon as the block wears off.

Another more frequent side effect of the interscalene block is the additional numbing of a nerve that goes to the diaphragm, a breathing muscle in the chest. This may cause a feeling of heavy breathing or even shortness of breath, but if present, most patients do not notice it. All that is usually required is to take deep and slow breaths until the condition rectifies itself, and to sit up so the abdominal organs do not press on the lungs. For this reason, an interscalene block may not be the best option for people with severe lung disease. Numbing some of the chest muscles that assist with breathing in people with lung disease can worsen breathing difficulties.

Minor bruising is not uncommon from this block injection and usually goes away in a couple of days. Infection or nerve injuries are always a potential complication, but are very rare.

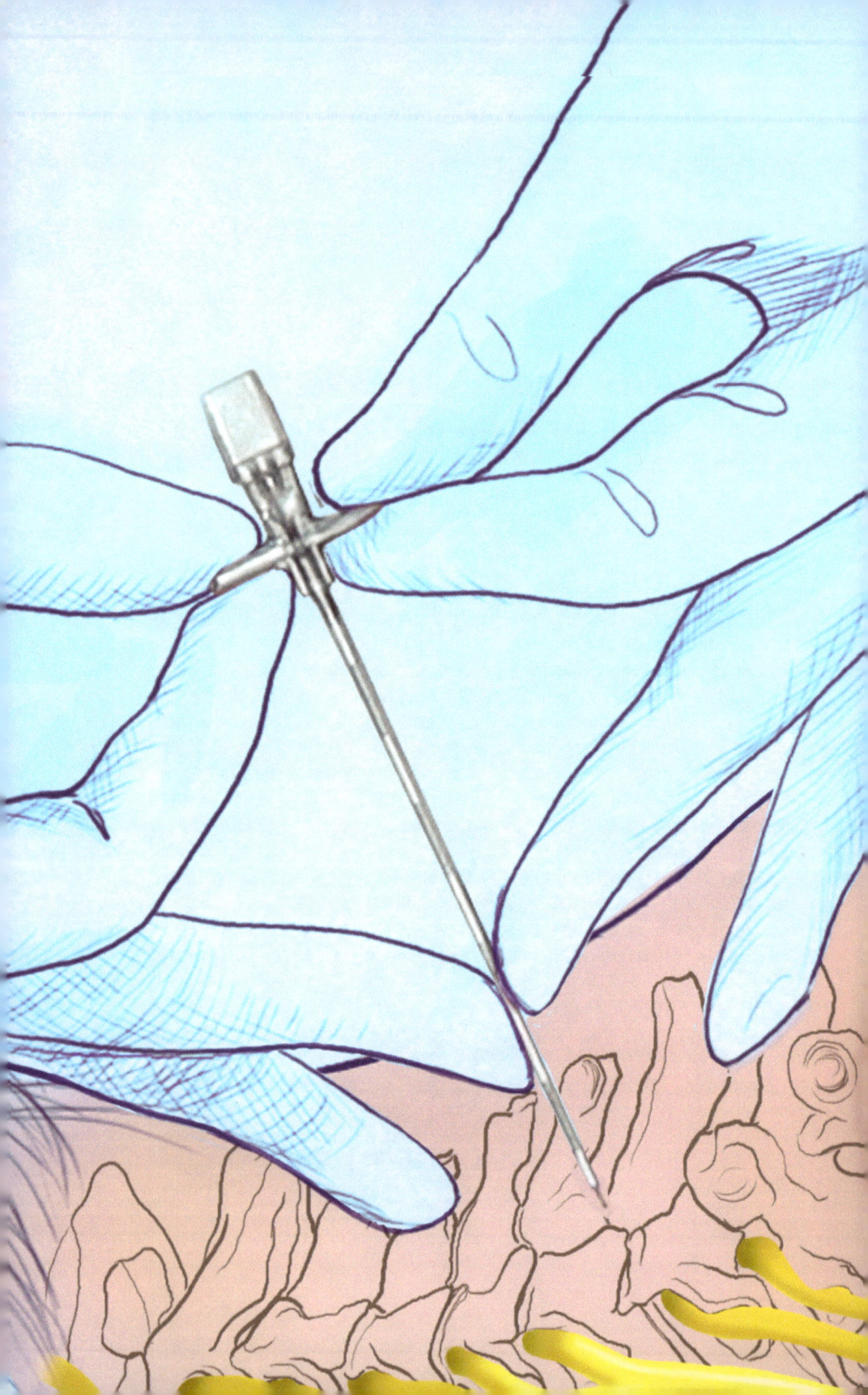

Cervical, Thoracic & Lumbar Paravertebral Blocks

33

[(para = adjacent or alongside;
vertebra = a bone segment of the spinal column)]

Paravertebral blocks can be used for surgery to the arm, elbow, wrist, shoulder, chest, abdomen, and upper legs. The block targets a space along the spine where multiple nerve fibers emerge from the spinal cord. In the right hands, these blocks are very safe and very effective. Local anesthetic agents injected into this space provides excellent post-operative pain control. This is especially important for patients planning to have physical therapy after surgery.

The needle insertion point varies depending on the type of surgery to be performed, but will be either to the right or left of the spinal column. A cervical paravertebral block is performed on the very upper back or lower neck, while thoracic paravertebral block is done in the chest (or thoracic) area and lumbar paravertebral in the lower back (or lumbar) area. They are all basically the same and the level depends on the type of surgery planned. For example, for shoulder surgery a cervical paravertebral block would be done, for breast surgery and chest and upper abdominal surgery a thoracic paravertebral block will be done and for hip and lower extremity surgery a lumbar paravertebral block.

What are the risks of paravertebral blocks?

The side effects associated with cervical paravertebral blocks are related to numbing the other nerves of the arm, shoulder, and neck. Horner's syndrome is a temporary condition after a paravertebral block in which individuals have unequal pupils and sometimes a slight drooping of one eyelid. People sometimes also get mild hoarseness from the block. This happens because a branch of the nerve running to the vocal cords is numbed too. Patients might also experience the feeling of a stuffy nose. Although unwanted, these are the usual effects of a working nerve block and not dangerous complications.

Under very rare circumstances, a tissue layer surrounding the lung, the pleura, can be punctured while performing a thoracic paravertebral block, resulting in air entering the space between the pleura and the lung. The injury causes a condition known as a pneumothorax. The symptoms of a pneumothorax include shortness of breath and sometimes chest pain on the affected side. These symptoms can develop several hours after the block and could potentially occur after the patient is home from surgery. If patients experience any problems with their breathing, then they should call the hospital immediately, visit a local emergency department, or call 911.

For all paravertebral blocks, the risk of infection, although rare, increases with the time that the catheter is left in. Patients should report any pain, discharge or redness from the puncture site, fever, and weakness or numbness not explained by a recent injection of local anesthetic immediately to a nurse or physician.

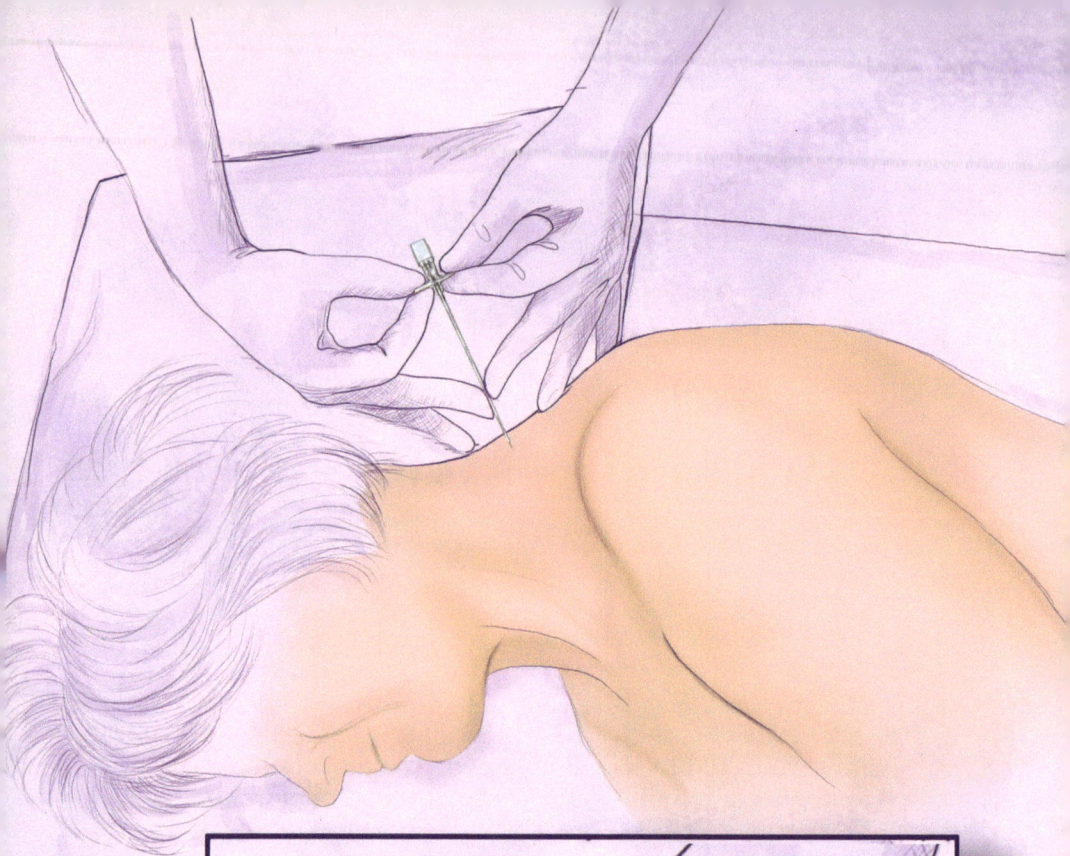
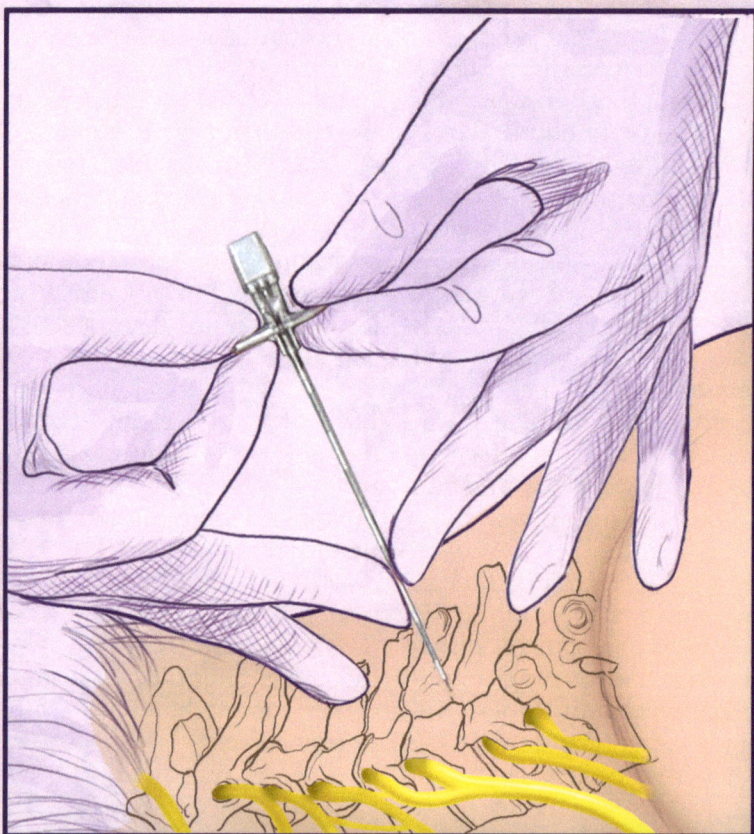

Bryson©

The Cervical Paravertebral Block

[(para = adjacent or alongside;

vertebra = a bone segment of the spinal column)]

37

A cervical paravertebral block is performed on the very upper back or lower neck. Although sedation isn't routinely required, medications are always available to help patients relax and to prevent any discomfort from the nerve block procedure. Patients having a cervical paravertebral block are positioned on their side, or sitting with the head slightly bent forward. After carefully cleaning the skin with antiseptic soap, the anesthesiologist will use a very fine needle to numb the skin and underlying tissue. This is not uncomfortable or painful. The local anesthetic will quickly numb the area, making the rest of the procedure more comfortable. After the injection, patients should only feel pressure as the anesthesiologist works. A specialized needle will then be used to locate and inject medication for the paravertebral nerve block. Patients will likely experience a mild muscle contraction from the nerve stimulator if used, but the so-called "Dual technique" where ultrasound- and nerve stimulator-guidance is used is the popular way of performing this block. If a nerve stimulator is also used, it is normal to feel the muscle twitches. These are similar to your eye twitching, only it is in your upper arm muscles. You cannot control it and it should not be uncomfortable or painful. If a continuous infusion is planned for post-operative pain control, a fine catheter will be inserted before the special needle is withdrawn. A single injection of anesthetic medication can provide pain relief for up to 8 hours. The continuous infusion catheter can deliver pain-relieving medication for as long as the catheter and pump are needed.

FIGURE 4:
Cervical paravertebral block.
Patient is lying on his/her side
or can be sitting up.

Risks of cervical paravertebral blocks

38

A cervical paravertebral block will cause the arm and shoulder to become numb. Superficial nerves, especially in the arm, are vulnerable to injury because patients will not feel any pressure on these nerves. The surgical team will take special precautions when positioning patients during surgery. After surgery, patients are fitted with a padded arm sling and provided with specific instructions on preventing accidental nerve injury. Special care should be taken to protect the elbow or "funny bone" area of the arm. The ulnar nerve in this area of the arm can easily be injured.

The Thoracic Paravertebral Block

39

Thoracic paravertebral blocks are commonly done for major breast surgery or unilateral (one-sided) chest or upper abdominal surgery. The procedure is essentially similar to the cervical paravertebral block, just in the thoracic or chest area, and potential complications include pneumothorax (lung collapse), and all the potential complications associated with epidural block.

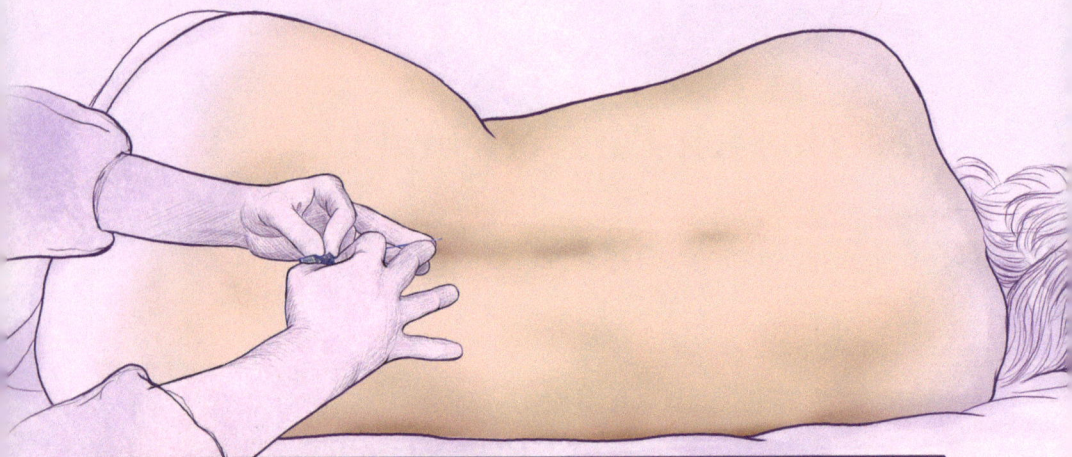

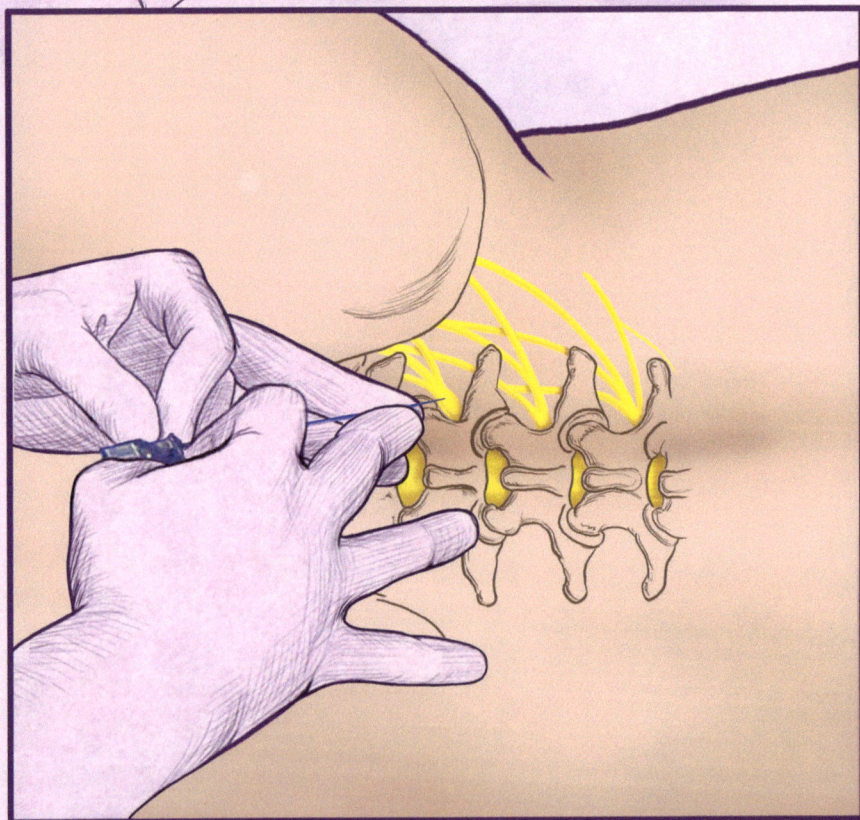

BRYSON©

The Lumbar Paravertebral Block

41

Lumbar paravertebral block is also sometimes called Psoas Compartment Block or Lumbar Plexus block. It essentially performed the same as the cervical paravertebral block, just in the lumbar region and for lower limb surgery. Potential problems are similar to those associated with epidural block and also bleeding and kidney damage have been described.

FIGURE 5:
Lumbar paravertebral block.
Patient is lying on his/her side
or can be sitting up.

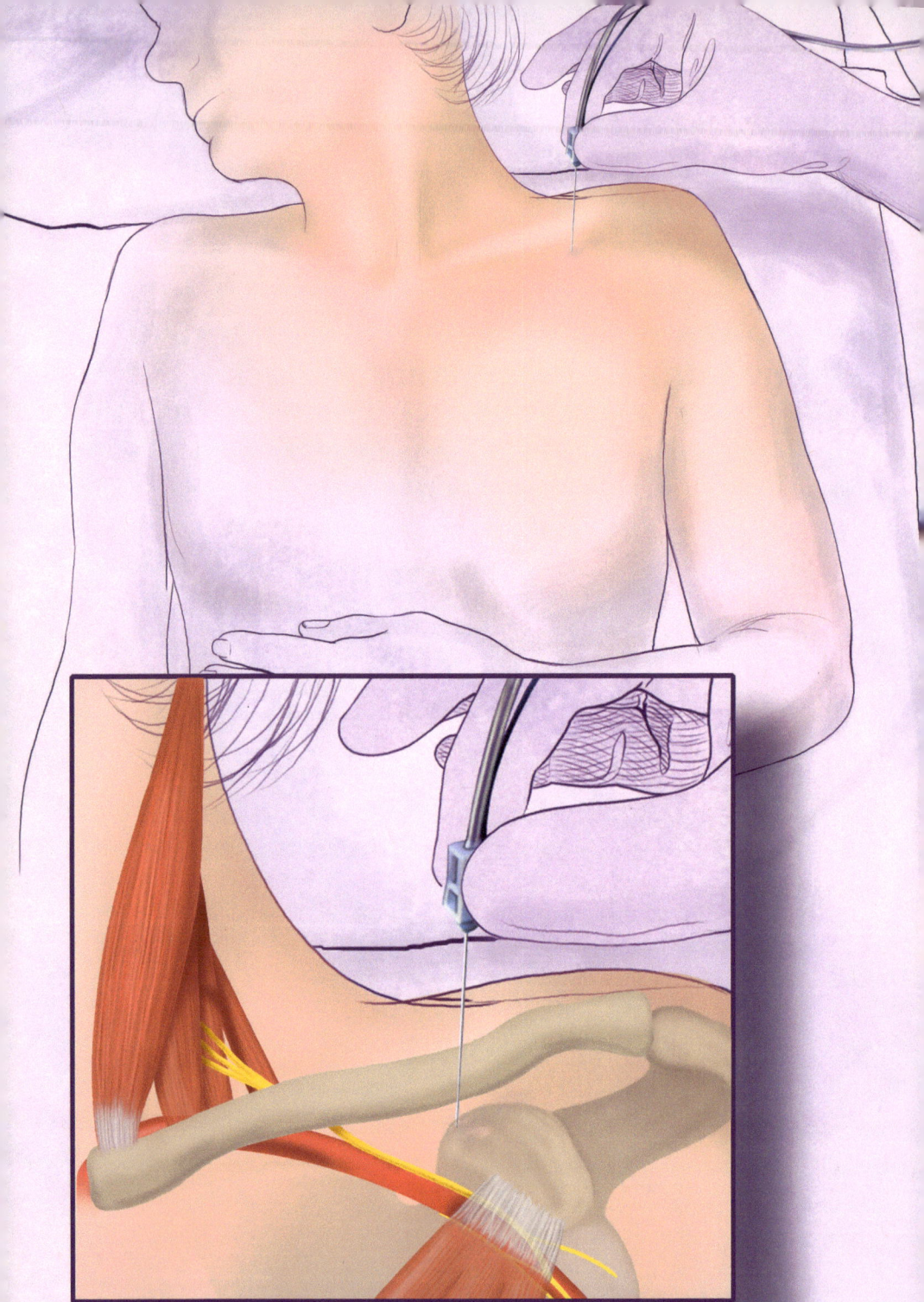

BRYSON©

Supraclavicular & Infraclavicular Nerve Blocks

43

**[supra = above; infra = below;
clavicular = refers to the collarbone]**

Supraclavicular and infraclavicular are words used to identify different anatomical approaches to the same bundle of nerves called the brachial plexus. This bundle of nerves is found on the upper chest above and below the collarbone, or clavicle. The supraclavicular approach is slightly above the collarbone, and the infraclavicular approach below the collarbone. Either approach can provide a block ideally suited as the sole anesthetic for the surgical procedure and for relief of post-operative pain following surgery to the arm, elbow, wrist, or hand.

FIGURE 6:
*Infraclavicular block.
Supraclavicular block is similar, but the
needle entry is above the clavicle.*

A combination of blocks is especially useful for surgery involving the use of a tourniquet on the upper arm. Two separate blocks are required to numb the different nerves that supply sensation to the upper arm. Tourniquets are useful during surgery because they compress blood vessels and temporarily stop blood flow to the arm. Supraclavicular or infraclavicular blocks provide complete numbness from the upper arm to the fingertips, but do not typically include the shoulder.

For this block, patients are positioned on their back. After carefully cleaning the skin with antiseptic soap, the anesthesiologist will use a very fine needle to numb the skin and underlying tissue. This block is not uncomfortable or painful. The local anesthetic will quickly numb the area, making the rest of the procedure more comfortable. After the injection, patients should only feel pressure as the anesthesiologist works. A specialized needle will then be used to locate and inject medication for the nerve block. These two blocks are almost entirely done with ultrasound-guidance only. If, in the rare occasions that a nerve stimulator is also used, patients will likely experience a very mild sensation or muscle contraction running down the arm from the nerve stimulator, and their fingers or hands should move similar to the eye twitching. You cannot control this is normal and should not be painful or uncomfortable. If a continuous infusion is planned for post-operative pain control, a fine catheter will be inserted before the special needle is withdrawn. A single injection of anesthetic medication can provide pain relief for up to 8 hours. The continuous infusion catheter can deliver pain-relieving medication for as long as the catheter and pump are needed.

Risks of supraclavicular or infraclavicular blocks

Under very rare circumstances, a tissue layer surrounding the lung, the pleura, can be punctured while performing the block, resulting in air entering the space between the pleura and the lung. This is extremely rare if ultrasound-guidance is used, but may cause a condition known as a pneumothorax. The symptoms of a pneumothorax include shortness of breath and sometimes chest pain on the affected side. These symptoms can develop several hours after the block, and could potentially occur after patients are home from surgery. If patients experience any problems with their breathing, then they should call the hospital immediately, visit a local emergency department, or call 911.

A supraclavicular or infraclavicular block will cause the arm to become numb. Superficial nerves, especially in the arm, are vulnerable to injury because patients will not feel any pressure on these nerves. The surgical team will take special precautions when positioning the patient during surgery. After surgery, patients are fitted with a padded arm sling and provided with specific instructions on preventing accidental nerve injury. Special care should be taken to protect the elbow or "funny bone" area of the arm. The ulnar nerve in this area of the arm can easily be injured.

The risk of infection, although rare, increases with the time that the catheter is left in. Patients should report any pain, discharge from the puncture site, fever, and weakness or numbness not explained by a recent injection of local anesthetic immediately to a nurse or physician.

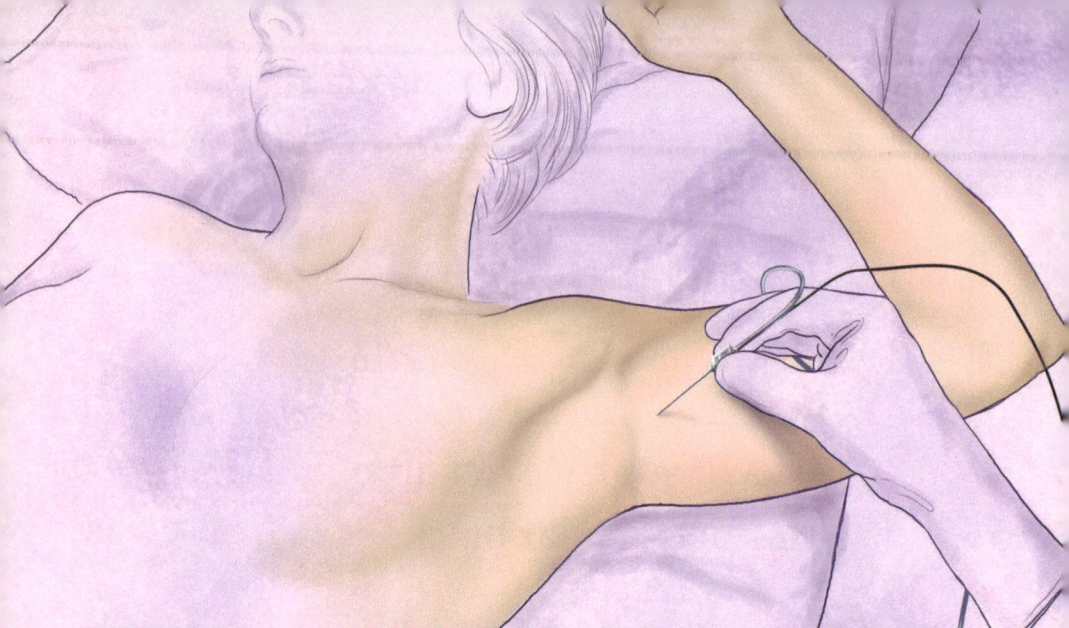

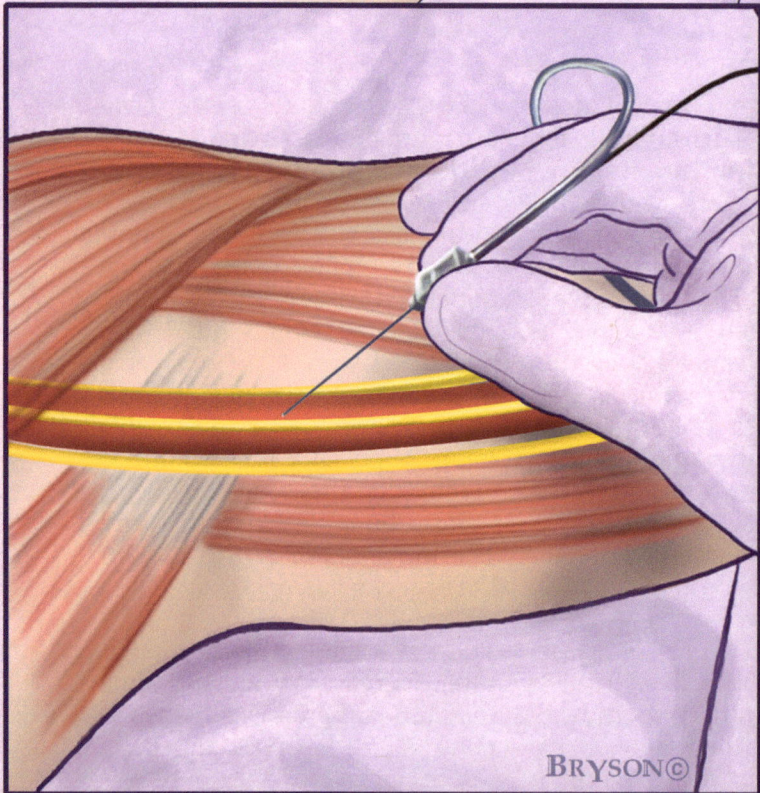

BRYSON©

Axillary Blocks
[Axilla = underarm]

The axillary nerve block is used for hand, wrist, forearm, and elbow surgery.

FIGURE7::
Axillary block.

48

For this block, patients are positioned on their back, arm extended away from the body and the elbow bent. After carefully cleaning the skin with antiseptic soap, the anesthesiologist will use a very fine needle to numb the skin and underlying tissue in the axilla. This block is not uncomfortable or painful. The local anesthetic will quickly numb the area, making the rest of the procedure more comfortable. After the injection, patients should only feel pressure as the anesthesiologist works. A special needle will be used to locate and inject medication for the nerve block. This block is almost always done with ultrasound-guidance only, but if nerve stimulation is also used, you will likely experience a very mild sensation or muscle contraction running down the arm from the nerve stimulator. If a continuous infusion is planned for post-operative pain control, a fine catheter will be inserted before the special needle is withdrawn. A single injection of anesthetic medication can provide pain relief for up to 8 hours. The continuous infusion catheter can deliver pain-relieving medication for as long as the catheter and pump are needed.

What Are The Risks Of Axillary Blocks?

Axillary blocks require a relatively large dose of anesthetic medications to fully numb the lower arm. Occasionally, the numbing effect of the block will be patchy, leaving surfaces of the hand and lower arm sensitive.

An axillary block may not be possible if patients are unable to position their arm away from their body with the elbow bent.

Side effects from the anesthetic medications are of special concern with axillary blocks. The target nerve bundles for this block lie in close proximity to a large blood vessel supplying the arm, the axillary artery. Possible complications include absorption of the medication into the axillary artery and/or injury to the artery, resulting in bleeding.

The presence of hair and moisture in the axilla may increase the risk of infection. The longer a continuous catheter is left in, the greater the risk. Patients should report any pain, discharge from the puncture site, fever, and weakness or numbness not explained by a recent injection of local anesthetic immediately to a nurse or physician.

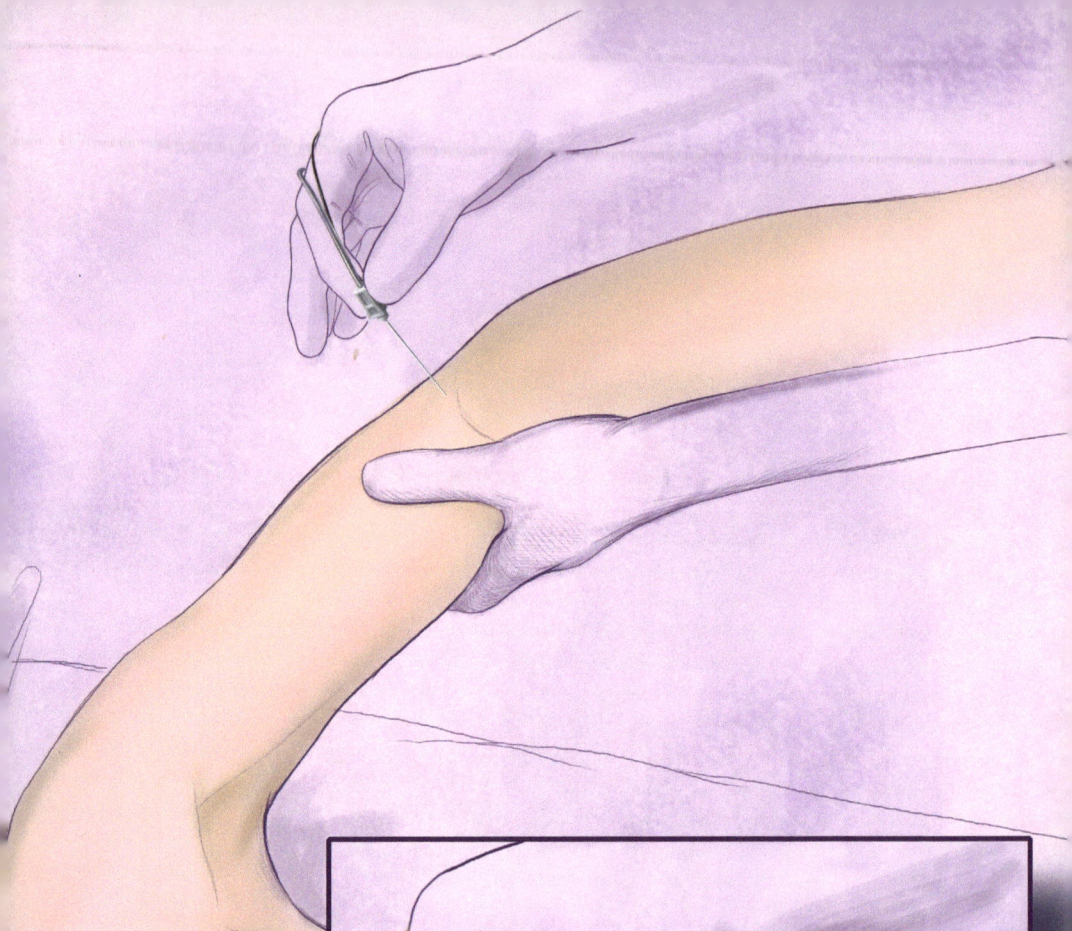

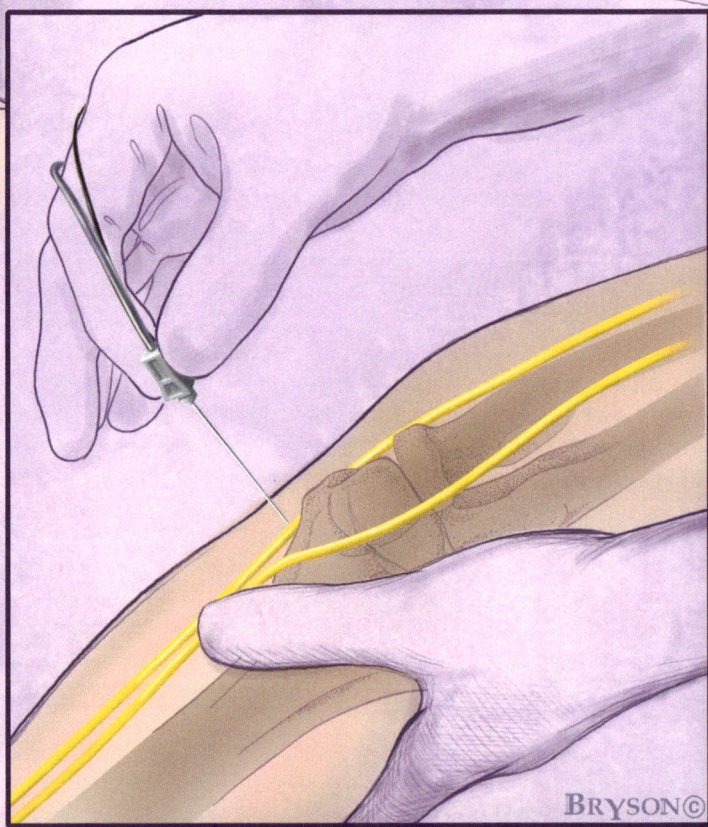

BRYSON©

Elbow Blocks

Four nerves supply sensation to the lower arm and hand. These are the ulna, radial, median and musculocutaneous nerves.

FIGURE 8:
Elbow block.

52

An elbow block requires shots of local anesthetic at three separate locations around the elbow. Elbow blocks are sometimes used for hand surgeries and can also provide additional numbness from an incomplete axillary, infraclavicular, or supraclavicular block. For an elbow block, patients are positioned on their back with the arm extended away from the body. After cleaning the skin with antiseptic soap, the anesthesiologist will use a fine needle to inject local anesthetic. Ultrasound-guidance is almost always used for this block and the anesthesiologist may reposition the arm after each injection. Elbow blocks can provide pain relief for 6 to 8 hours.

What are the risks of elbow blocks?

Elbow blocks will not provide numbness to the forearm, so the block's usefulness is limited to hand surgery. Because the nerves are found at three different places in the elbow, a continuous catheter for long-term pain management cannot be used.

The main concerns of an elbow block include accidental injection of local anesthetic into a blood vessel or injection of too much medication, leading to nerve compression and injury. The anesthesiologist will take precautions to minimize the risks. Other complications like permanent nerve damage, bleeding, or infection are very rare but possible.

As with all blocks to an arm or leg, patients will need to take special care of the hand following surgery until sensation fully returns. Depending on the medications used, the hand and forearm may remain numb for 24 hours or longer. Patients usually wear an arm sling after surgery to support and protect the hand.

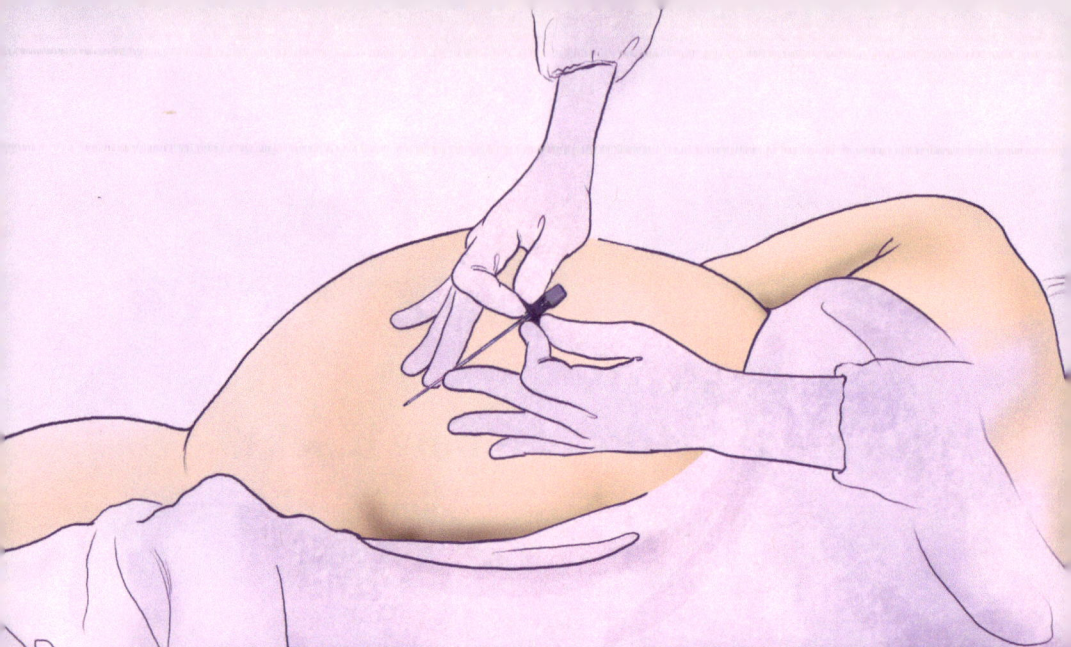

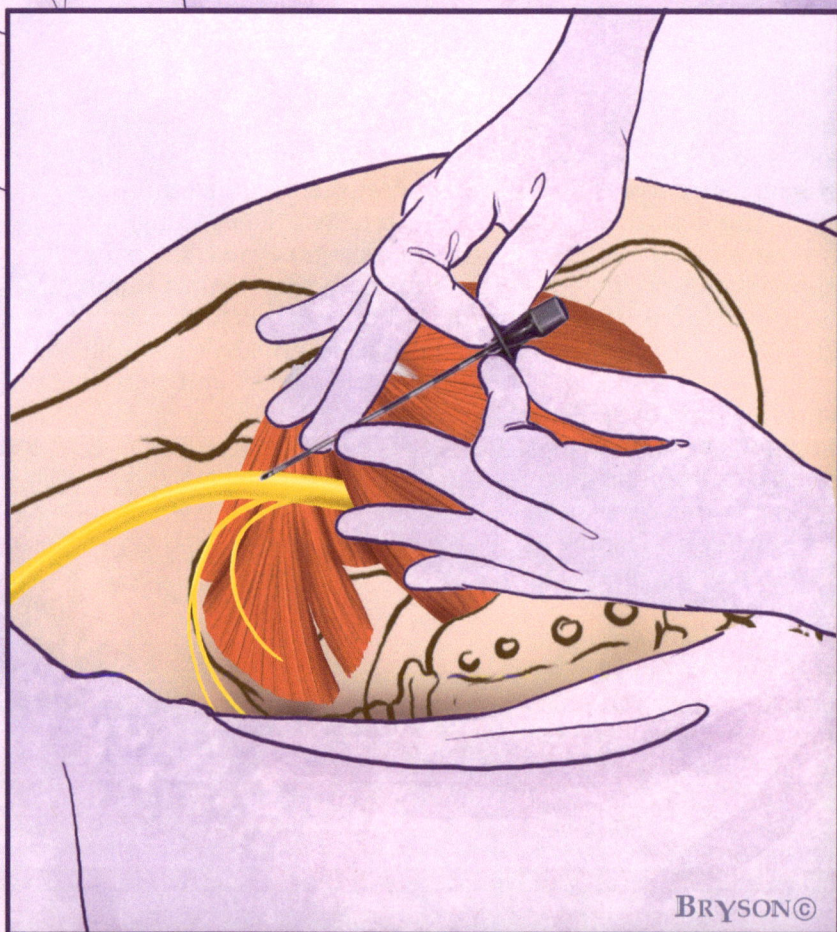

Sciatic Nerve Blocks
[Sciatic = hip]

Sciatic nerve blocks are used for surgery to the back part of the upper leg, back of the knee and most of the lower leg, foot and ankle. The sciatic nerve is the largest and longest nerve in the body. Anesthetic blocks to the sciatic nerve tend to last longer than other nerve blocks. Continuous sciatic nerve blocks are usually reserved for major foot and ankle surgery, such as ankle reconstruction.

FIGURE 9A:
Subgluteal approach to sciatic nerve block with patient on his/her side and hip slightly flexed.

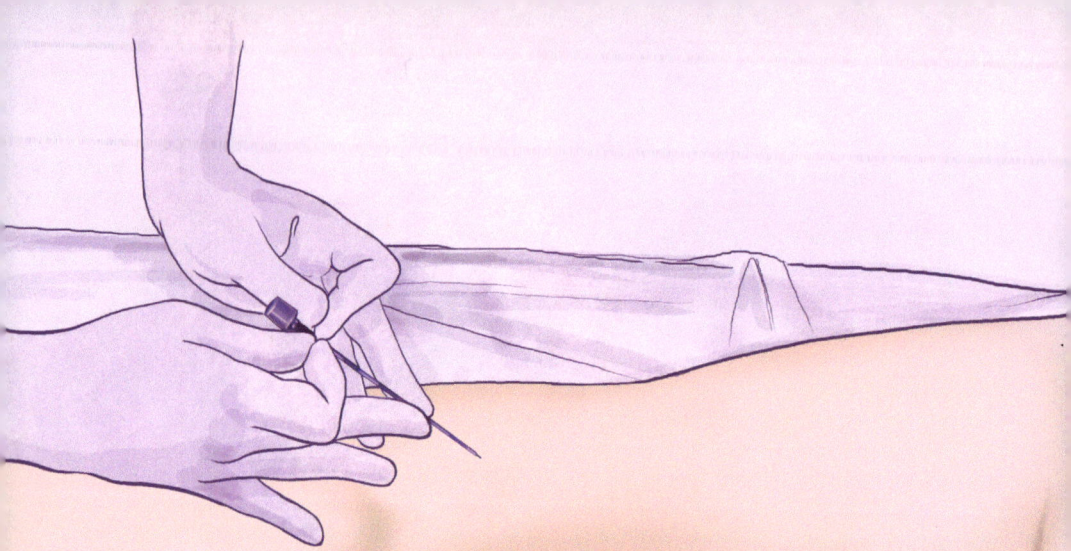

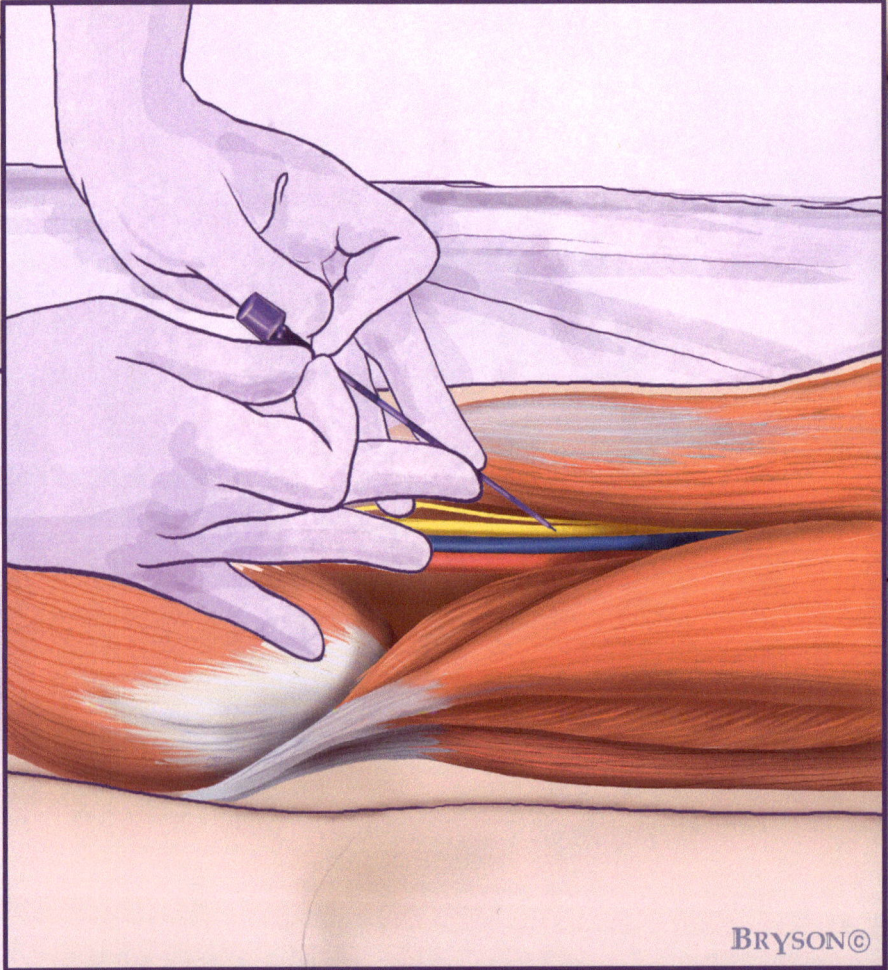

BRYSON©

Severe injury, obesity or illnesses like arthritis often limit movement or prevent individuals from lying comfortably in certain positions. Anesthesiologists have found several locations along the hip and upper leg to block the sciatic nerve. Patient positioning for the nerve block procedure will depend on the approach used.

Needle insertion for a posterior, or "Labat," sciatic nerve block is about halfway down the buttock. For this approach, patients are positioned on their non-surgical side with the upper leg bent at the knee and resting over the lower leg. The Labat approach is one of the older types of sciatic nerve blocks still in limited use.

The "Winnie" sciatic nerve block is a modified version of the Labat block. Needle insertion is in a different area of the buttock. Patients are positioned on their non-surgical side with the upper leg bent

FIGURE 9B:
Popliteal approach to the sciatic nerve block.

at the knee and resting over the lower leg.

Needle insertion for a parasacral sciatic nerve block is along the outer hip, slightly below the waistline. For this approach, patients are positioned on their non-surgical side, almost on their stomach. The upper leg will be bent at the hip and knee.

Needle insertion for a subgluteal sciatic nerve block is along the skin fold separating the buttock from the leg (Figure 9a). For this block, patients are usually positioned on their non-surgical side with the upper leg bent at the knee and resting over the lower leg, or on their stomach. This is a common approach for continuous sciatic nerve blocks.

Needle insertion for a lateral sciatic nerve block is on the outer part of the leg midway down the thigh. The lateral approach can be used on patients lying on their back or side.

Needle insertion for a popliteal sciatic nerve block is behind the knee a couple of inches up from the skin fold (Figure 9b) For a popliteal block, patients will need to lie on their sides or stomach. This is the most commonly used approach to the sciatic nerve. Since nerve fibers branch with increasing frequency farther down the leg, it is possible to miss nerve fibers with a popliteal block, leaving only part of the lower leg numb.

The procedures for a single-injection or continuous catheter insertion are the same, regardless of the approach used. Any hair around the needle entry site will be removed, and then the skin will be cleaned with antiseptic soap. The anesthesiologist will use a fine needle to inject local anesthetic into the skin and underlying tissues. This first shot is the most uncomfortable part of the procedure, but should not be painful. The local anesthetic will quickly numb the area, making the rest of the procedure more comfortable. After the injection, patients should only feel pressure as the anesthesiologist works. For most of the approaches to the sciatic nerve ultrasound and nerve stimulator-guidance are used; the so-called "Dual Technique" but some anesthesiologists favor ultrasound-guidance while other favor nerve stimulator-guidance. It does not matter, because both are effective and safe. A specialized needle will be used to locate and inject medication for the nerve block. If nerve stimulation is used, you may experience a sensation or muscle contraction running down the leg from the nerve stimulator used to locate the nerve. If a continuous infusion is planned for post-operative pain control, a fine catheter will be inserted before the special needle is withdrawn.

What are the risks of sciatic nerve blocks?

A sciatic nerve block alone will not provide complete numbness to the lower leg. It's almost always necessary to block other nerves in the leg, such as the femoral nerve, or its terminal branch that goes to the inner side of the lower leg, the saphenous nerve as well. The risks associated with a sciatic nerve block include accidental injection of local anesthetic into a blood vessel or injection of too much medication, leading to nerve compression and injury. This is extremely rare and unheard of in most approaches to the sciatic nerve. The Labat and Winnie approaches are more prone to this complication. The anesthesiologist will take precautions to minimize risk. Mild bruising at the needle entry site is fairly common and usually resolves in a couple of days. Other complications like permanent nerve damage or infection are rare but possible.

As with all blocks to an arm or leg, patients will need to take special care of the leg following surgery until sensation fully returns. The common peroneal nerve, as it curves around the bone (fibula) on the outside of the lower leg, just below the knee, is especially at risk. Depending on the medications used, the leg may remain numb for 24 hours or longer.

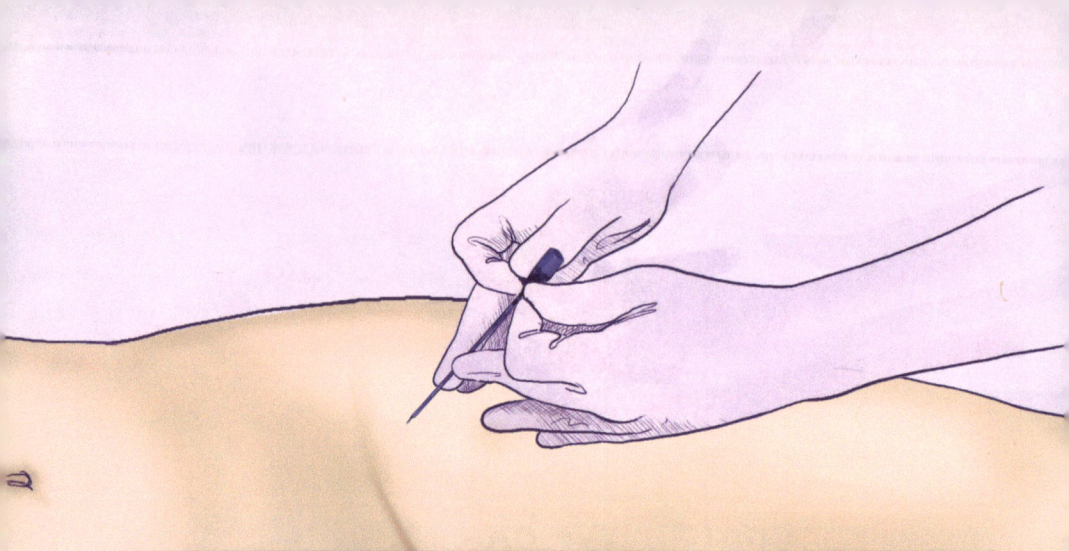

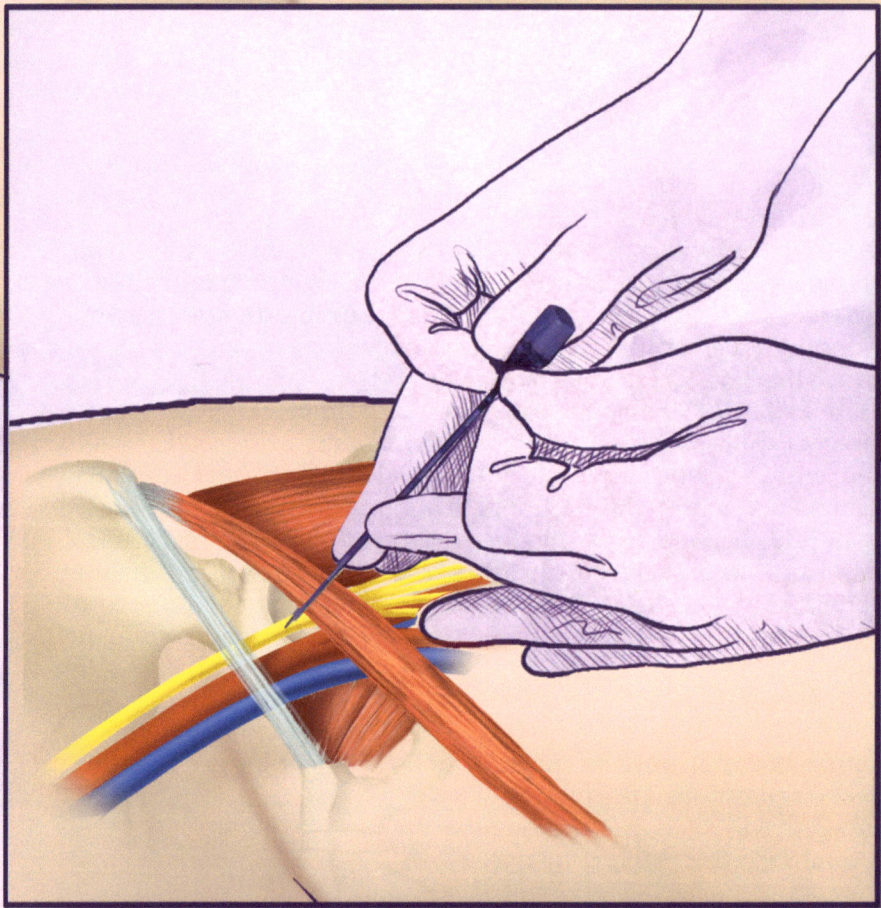

BRYSON

Femoral Nerve Blocks
[Femur = thigh bone]

The leg is supplied with many nerves that transmit sensation and movement signals. The femoral nerve transmits signals to and from much of the front and sides of the thigh, knee, and lower leg. The femoral nerve lies relatively close to the skin as it travels through the groin area down the leg. The femoral artery is in close proximity to this nerve. Femoral nerve blocks are used for surgery on the thigh, hip, knee, and inner areas of the lower leg. A second type of nerve block, the sciatic nerve block, is usually required to fully numb the lower leg.

FIGURE 10::
Femoral nerve block with patient in the supine position.

The needle insertion point for this block is in, below or above the inguinal skin fold that separates the leg from the trunk of body. Patients are positioned on their back for the block. Any hair in this area will be shaved. The skin around the needle entry site will be cleaned with antiseptic soap. After the skin and tissues under the skin are numbed thoroughly with a very fine needle, a special needle will be inserted into the skin. Ultrasound and nerve stimulator guidance in combination or separately are used for this block.

Patients should feel pressure in the area of the needle insertion, but no pain. If nerve stimulation is used, patients will likely experience a very mild sensation or muscle contraction running down their leg from the nerve stimulator used to locate the nerve. If a continuous infusion is planned for post-operative pain control, a fine catheter will be inserted before the special needle is withdrawn.

What are the risks of femoral nerve blocks?

The risks associated with a femoral nerve block include accidental injection of local anesthetic into a blood vessel or injection of too much medication, leading to nerve compression and injury. This complication is extremely rare. The anesthesiologist will take precautions to minimize risk. Mild bruising at the needle entry site is fairly common and usually resolves in a few days. Other complications such as permanent nerve damage is very rare but possible.

The longer a continuous femoral catheter is left in, the greater the risk of infection. Patients should report any pain, discharge from the puncture site, fever, and weakness or numbness not explained by a recent injection of local anesthetic immediately to a nurse or physician.

As with all blocks to an arm or leg, patients will need to take special care of the leg following surgery until sensation fully returns. Depending on the medications used, the leg may remain numb for 12 hours or longer.

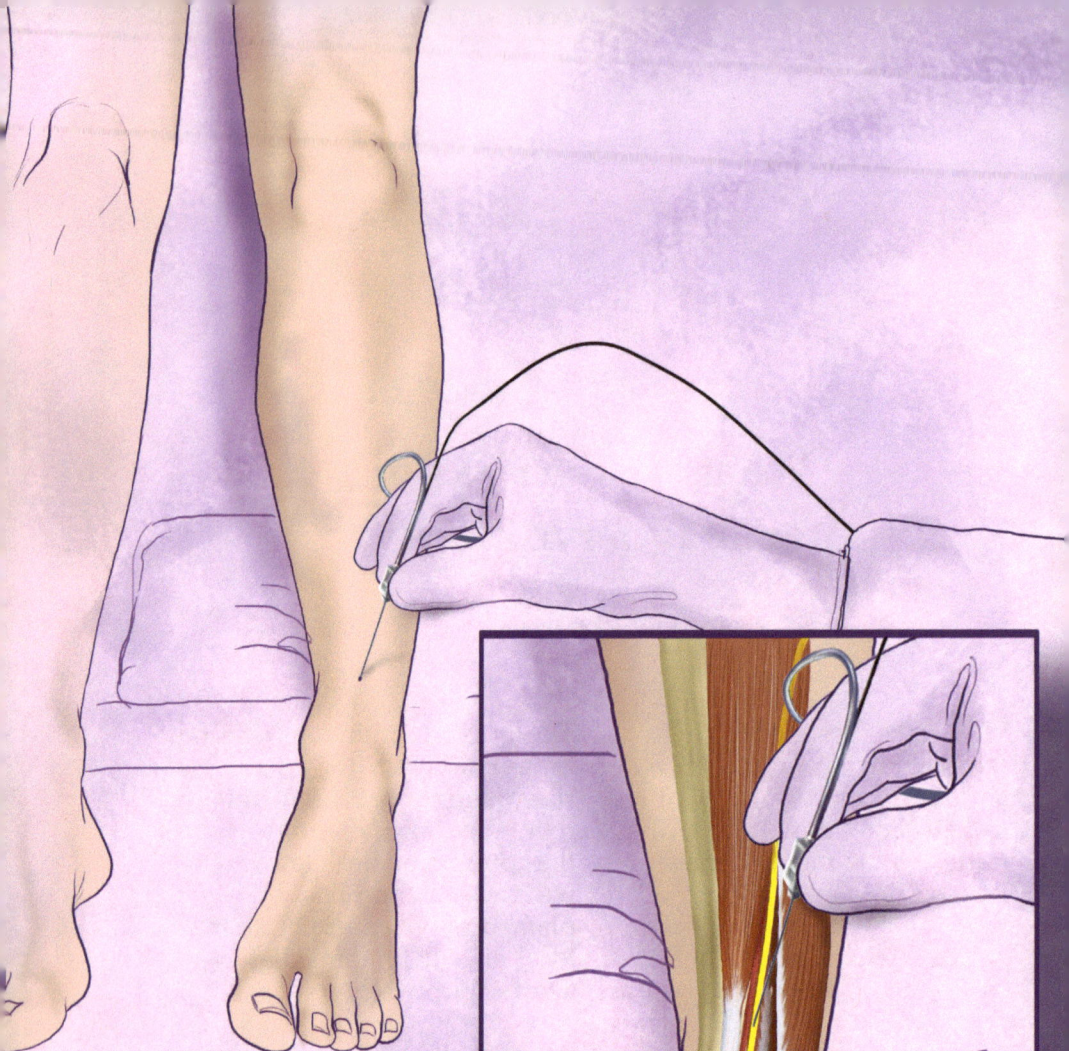

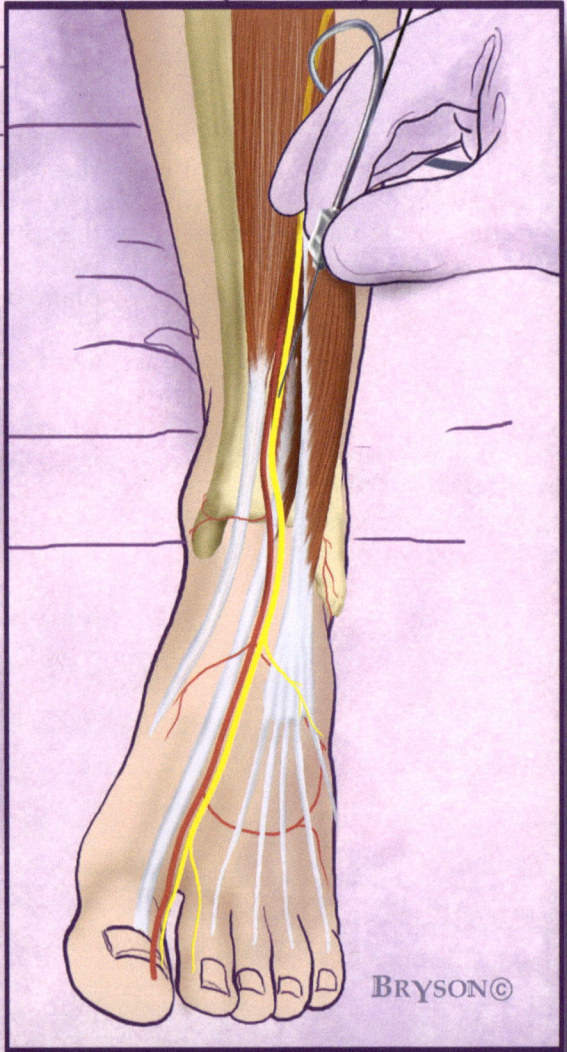

BRYSON©

Ankle Blocks

65

An ankle block is a common type of block used for foot surgery. It is not a popular block if the skin around the ankle is swollen or scarred in any way. Five separate nerve fibers supply sensation to the foot and control movement. Depending upon the anesthetic drug used, injections at various points around the ankle can provide numbing pain relief for 6 to 18 hours.

FIGURE 11:
Ankle block.

For an ankle block, patients are positioned on their back. The anesthesiologist will rotate the foot as needed to reach the injection sites. This block requires two to five different injections of medication into the ankle. Medications will be available to help patients relax and to prevent any discomfort from the nerve block procedure. After carefully cleaning the foot and ankle with antiseptic soap, the anesthesiologist will use a fine needle to inject numbing medication. It usually takes 10 to 20 minutes for the medication to fully numb the foot. Ultrasound or nerve stimulation may be used to do this block, but most skilled practitioners use no aids, because this is such a superficial block. Only the nerve on the inside behind the ankle may be difficult to find without these aids.

What are the risks of ankle blocks?

Patients may experience mild pain from the injections of numbing medications. Minor bruising is not uncommon from the ankle block injections and usually goes away in a couple of days. Infection or nerve injuries are potential complications, but very rare following an ankle block.

The greatest concern following an ankle block is accidental injury following surgery. The foot may remain numb for 24 hours or longer. Patients having foot surgery usually wear a special shoe following the procedure. The shoe will keep the foot dressing clean and dry and protect the skin from injury. Since the foot will not have sensation to heat or cold, patients should not use a heating pad or ice packs unless specifically instructed by the doctor.

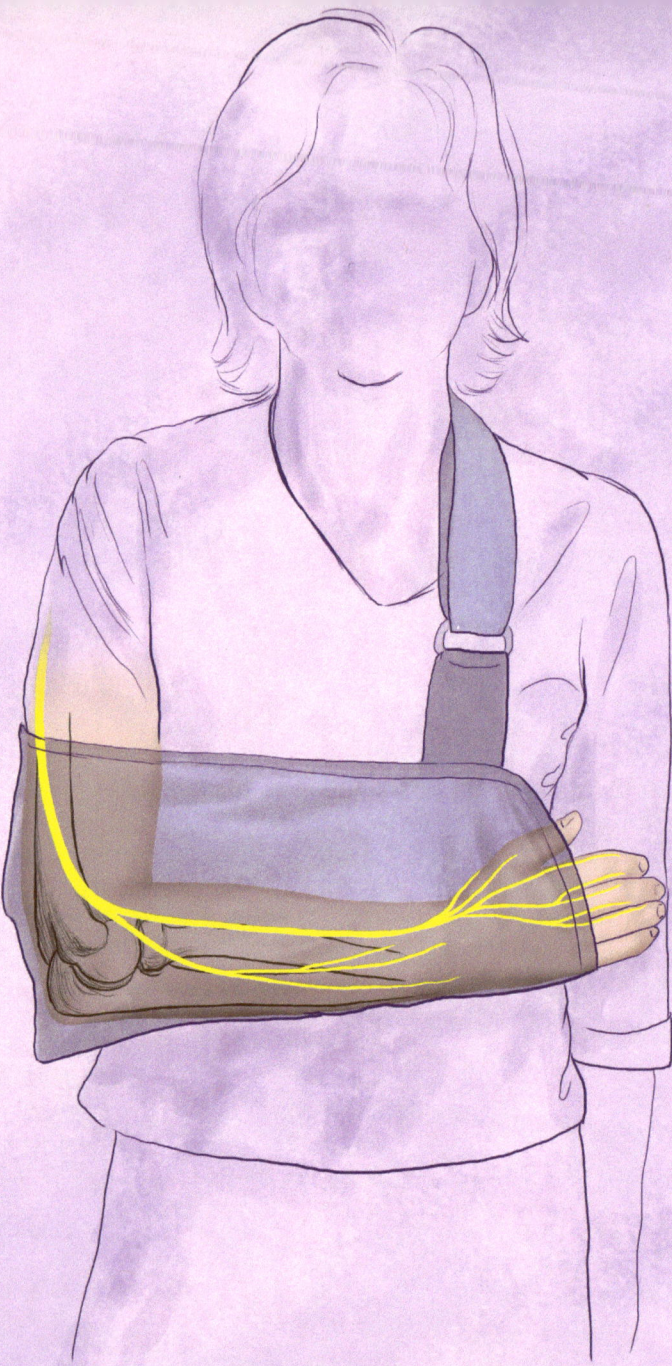

BRYSON©

Precautions

Patients should not attempt to walk without crutches and assistance after any block of the lower extremity. Unassisted walking may result in falls and serious injury.

Patients should avoid using ice packs or heating pads on numb limbs. They will not be able to feel excessive heat or cold applied to the area, which can result in skin damage. Likewise, patients will also not be able to feel a bump to the limb, and this can lead to injury; it is essential to check for any signs of infection (warmness, redness, swelling) regularly.

FIGURE 12A:
Correct sling fit in standing patient.

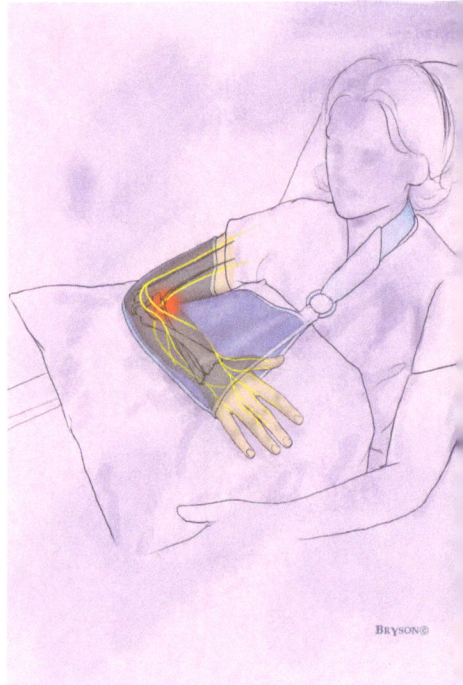

70

If an arm sling is fitted, then proper fitting must be ensured. It is essential that at all times the elbow is bent 90 degrees or more (Figure 12a). The sling should not be adjusted to angles greater than 90 degrees (Figure 12b), since this may cause pressure on the radial nerve where it curls around the midsection of the humerus, the bone in the upper arm.

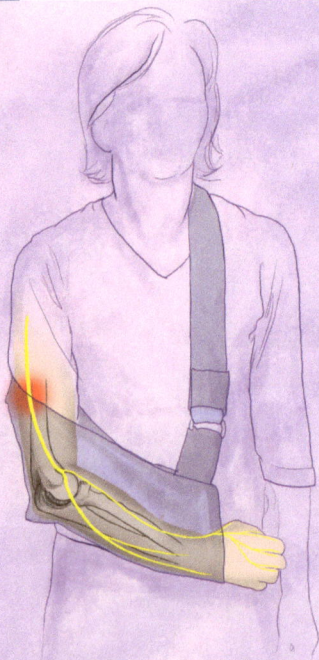

While the arm is numbed, elbow should always be protected with a soft pillow (Figure 12c). The ulnar nerve, or "funny bone," behind the elbow can be exposed to pressure, and it can be damaged. The pressure cannot be felt, and patients will not know about it while their arm is numbed. This pressure can severely damage this nerve. Special care should be taken when sleeping (see Fig. 12c).

FIGURE 12B (left):
Incorrect arm sling fit in standing patient. Note pressure on the nerve in the upper arm.

FIGURE 12C (above):
Arm on pillows protecting the ulnar nerve indicated by the red area.

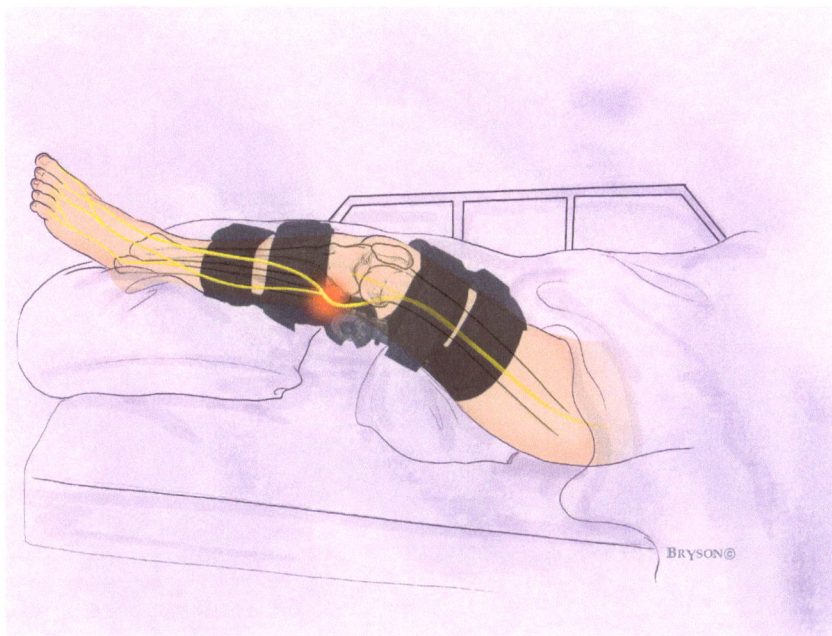

71

Similarly, if the leg is numbed, the area just below the knee should be ensured to be free from any pressure. One should always be able to fit two fingers between the cast (or brace) and any bony parts. This is especially true where the common peroneal nerve is found on the outside of the leg. If a lower leg cast is fitted or a knee brace is applied, patients should never lie on the side that has been operated upon. The lower leg should be supported on soft pillows and the area about 6 inches above and 6 inches below the

knee should be protected and free of any pressure, especially when the patient is sleeping (Figure 13).

Always evaluate the toes and fingers for color and swelling. The color should be the same as the other foot and hand. There should not be blue discoloration or swelling. If patients have any doubt, then they should ask a healthcare provider to evaluate this, go to the local emergency room, or call 911. Any abnormal redness, discharge or bleeding from catheter sites should be immediately reported, as well as any unexpected symptom or sign, such as unexplained pain, swelling, or blue or red discoloration.

FIGURE 13:
Leg in brace. Be sure to protect the
common peroneal nerve, indicated by the red area.

72

Management Of Continuous Blocks
At Home

Continuous infusions allow people to return home much faster after surgery and avoid the use of opioid medication to a large extend. It is becoming more and more popular. The continuous infusion not only provides better pain control, but also has fewer side effects than traditional medications for pain taken by mouth, such as opiates. Planning for home care will begin when the surgery is scheduled or shortly after the surgery, while the patient is still in the hospital. Anesthesiology nurses will provide information to patients and their families about the catheter and pump, and they will also assist with home nursing care arrangements. After discharge from the hospital, a visiting nurse checks on the patient at home every day until the visits are no longer needed or someone from the team of the anesthesiologist will call you daily.

During their home continuous infusion therapy, patients can expect the following:

- A "mini-physical" exam will be conducted every day the catheter is in place.
- A nurse or physician will inspect the skin around the catheter entry site for signs of infection, such as tenderness, redness, and/or swelling.
- Patients will be asked questions about their ability to move the blocked arm or leg, and the degree of sensation they have.
- The catheter and pump will be inspected every day to make sure they are functioning properly.

After patients have been home for a day or two, the visiting nurse may call a few hours before the scheduled visit and ask patients to turn off the infusion pump. Turning off the infusion pump will allow patients and their nurses to determine if the continuous infusion therapy is still needed. Patients should not be alarmed if the pain returns. Patients can discuss options with the nurse, or contact the anesthesiologist's team. These options may include switching to oral pain-relieving medications or resuming the continuous infusion therapy.

Removal of the catheter at the end of continuous infusion therapy is a simple procedure done at home. The doctor may instruct patients to remove the catheter themselves and will guide them through the procedure, or the nurse will remove any dressings and tape used to secure the catheter and then slowly pull the catheter out. Removing the catheter should cause no pain or discomfort. It is very important that patients tell the nurse if they experience any shooting or sharp pain down the blocked arm or leg as the catheter is removed.

It takes 2 to 6 hours for normal sensation to fully return after the infusion has been stopped. If patients experience numbness, tingling or weakness lasting longer than 36 hours after the block or the infusion is stopped, the anesthesiologist should be notified. Also, the anesthesiologist should be informed if any signs of infection are observed; these include fever, redness, tenderness, pain, or drainage from the surgical wound or the catheter entry site.

74 Portable Infusion Pumps

Portable infusion pumps come in a variety of shapes and sizes. Most pumps run on batteries, and most are disposable A shoulder strap or fanny pack is usually provided to hold the portable pump. The pump's medication reservoir size varies from model to model, but is usually large enough to last for several days without a refill. Regardless of the model, all portable infusion pumps do the same thing: They are designed to provide a continuous infusion of local anesthetic through the catheter to the nerve. The infusion pump also allows patients to give themselves additional medication through the catheter for "break through" pain. Patients do not have to worry about overdosing or receiving too much medication because the pump has built-in safety features. The hospital staff or visiting nurses should ensure that patients have the information they need to feel at ease with the portable infusion pump.

Patients should treat the pump as they would any sensitive electrical device. The pump should be kept away from water and other liquids, and it should be protected from accidental bumps. In addition, it should be kept away from small children and pets. Remember, the pump is a patient's best friend during this time. The visiting nurse service should be available 24 hours a day to answer any questions or concerns.

Will there be additional costs for a nerve block?

It is very easy to overlook the cost of medical care until the day a bill arrives in the mail. Knowledge of insurance coverage and deductibles for services like a peripheral nerve block and/or a visiting nurse will help patients make informed decisions. After talking with the anesthesiologist, patients should check with the hospital billing office and their insurance provider for potential out-of-pocket expenses. A continuous peripheral nerve block catheter and visiting nurse support are a fraction of the costs associated with traditional hospital stays following surgery.

Where can healthcare providers go for more info?

76

Your local library and the Internet are good places to find additional information on peripheral nerve blocks. Patients should be sure to talk with their nurses, anesthesiologists, and surgeons. Together, healthcare providers and patients can come up with a plan tailored to meet each patient's needs. All the blocks, procedures, and precautions described in this booklet are available on the website: raeducation.com

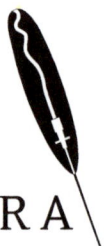

RA EDUCATION
regional anesthesia education
www.raeducation.com

www.ingramcontent.com/pod-product-compliance
Lightning Source LLC
Chambersburg PA
CBHW041716200326
41519CB00005B/271